Chapter one

Viva Smith had always been captivated by animals. Their beauty, their grace, and their mysterious ways fascinated her. Since she was a little girl, she dreamed of becoming a veterinarian, taking care of all creatures big and small. With her heart full of compassion and a genuine love for animals, she knew it was her calling in life.

One sunny afternoon, Viva and Derek her brother, returned from an enchanting visit to the local zoo. Viva's eyes sparkled with delight as she recounted the sightings of majestic lions, playful monkeys, and graceful dolphins to her brother. Her voice filled with enthusiasm, knowing she had found her true passion.

As they stepped through the front door of their cozy home, the aroma of comfort food greeted them. Their mother had lovingly prepared a warm and hearty meal for them. However, Viva's heart sank when she realized her favorite dish, a mouthwatering lasagna, which they all enjoyed.

Derek, on the other hand, had his own distractions. His love for video games had become an all-consuming hobby. The sound of pumping beats and the loud echoes of his gaming adventures echoed from his room, where he tirelessly spent hours perfecting his skills.

Viva turned to Derek, her eyes twinkling with affection. "Derek, my dear brother, could you please turn the volume down a notch? I have something exciting to share with you!"
Derek paused the game, slightly annoyed by the interruption. He glanced at Viva, her face practically glowing with anticipation. Unable to resist his sister's infectious enthusiasm, he obliged, turning down the volume to a more manageable level.

Viva took a deep breath, heart pounding with excitement. She began to tell Derek about her dream of becoming a veterinarian. She described the joy she felt at the zoo, observing how the keepers cared for the animals, nursing them back to health, and ensuring their well-being. Viva spoke passionately, her words brimming with compassion and dedication.

Derek listened intently, the annoyance in his eyes slowly giving way to wide-eyed curiosity. He had never seen Viva so animated, so full of purpose. Suddenly, the virtual battles and imagined victories seemed small in comparison to his sister's dream.
"You know, Viva," Derek said, his voice softer now, "I've always thought you were meant for something great. And if being a vet is what makes your heart sing, then I'll support you wholeheartedly."

Viva's eyes filled with tears of gratitude. She couldn't have asked for a better brother, someone who understood and embraced her dreams. She wrapped her arms around Derek, feeling an overwhelming sense of love and camaraderie.

With a renewed sense of purpose, Viva turned to her trusted companion, her phone, and began to research veterinary schools and the steps required to fulfill her dreams. She knew it would be a challenging journey, but she was ready to face it head-on.

Meanwhile, Derek felt a newfound motivation stirring within him. Inspired by his sister's passion, he realized that it was time to find his own path. He resolved to explore his interests, not only in video games but also in other creative pursuits. It was time for him to discover his own passion, just like Viva had.

They had lost their Dad at a young age, and it hasn't been easy for their single mom, Everyone knows the Smith family as kind and generous family, they never stopped caring for people, Mrs. Smith had taught her children how important giving is to the family, before her husband died, he used to take the family to help and support the orphanage Organization, although he is no longer with them, they still follow the step their father had set.

Mrs. Smith phone rang, she answered the phone, it's her late husband best friend Mr. Oliver, calling just to check up on her and her children. he asked about the house Mr. Smith was building before he died. Mrs.Smith Explained how difficult things had been since her husband died, she had not been able to get enough money to pay the workers that had been working on the house, before her husband pass away he promised to tell her something very important, but he never got the chance to.
Mr. Oliver understood the situation so he decided that he and his family would pay them a visit the next day.

After the call ended, Mrs. Smith Started preparing to go to work, she is the CEO of a insurance company and she has a very good reputation at her place of work. While leaving for work, she told her children she would be coming back late because she had plans to work extra time for extra money, so she would be able to pay some bills, as they drove off, she dropped them at school and left for work.

Viva knew her Mom would do anything for her and Derek, she admires how strong her Mother was; despite not having the support of her late father, Viva had promised her Mom that she will be a good girl and she will take good care of her and Derek.

The next day, the Oliver family consisting of Mr. and Mrs. Oliver, along with their daughter Cathy, decided to pay a visit to their close friends, Mrs. Smith and her children, Viva and Derek. They gathered at Mrs. Smith's cozy home, ready to spend a delightful afternoon together.

When Mr. Oliver arrived, he couldn't help but reminisce about his dear childhood friend, Mr. Smith, who had passed away many years ago. He fondly recalled the kindness and generosity that radiated from Mr. Smith's heart. Over a cup of tea, Mr. Oliver began sharing tales of their shared adventures and the memories they had created together. He spoke of how Mr. Smith used to lend a helping hand to anyone in need, always putting others before himself.

As Mr. Oliver delved into the conversation, he mentioned an unfinished house that Mr. Smith had been building before his unfortunate demise. The uncompleted structure stood as a symbol of their unfinished dreams and plans, but also as a poignant reminder of the wonderful man Mr. Smith had been.

Cathy, Derek, and Viva listened attentively to Mr. Oliver's stories, their eyes wide with curiosity and admiration for their fathers' friendship. They were captivated by the tales of kindness and the deep bond that had connected their families for many years.

In turn, Cathy, Derek, and Viva exchanged stories of their own. They spoke of their dreams for the future, sharing aspirations and ambitions that mirrored their fathers' friendship. It was a beautiful moment of connection, where the past met the present, and the younger generation carried on the legacy of friendship and compassion.

As the evening progressed, Mrs. Oliver and Mrs. Smith joined the conversation, sharing in the laughter and reminiscing about the times they had spent together. They marveled at the bond between their families that had stood the test of time.

Inspired by the tales of unfinished dreams and the enduring friendship between their parents, Cathy, Derek, and Viva made a pact. They promised to support each other in pursuing their dreams, just as their fathers had supported one another.

With renewed determination and a shared sense of purpose, the Oliver and Smith children understood the importance of kindness, friendship, and carrying forward the legacies of their fathers.

As the sun began to set, the Oliver and Smith families bid each other farewell, but the memory of their gathering lingered in their hearts. They knew that, no matter what the future held, the bond forged during their visit would forever remain strong.

In the following weeks and months, Cathy, Derek, and Viva stayed connected, supporting each other through both triumphs and challenges. They celebrated each other's achievements, offering words of encouragement and lending a helping hand whenever needed.

Inspired by her father's stories of Mr. Smith's kindness, Cathy began volunteering at a local charity, dedicating her time to helping those less fortunate. Derek discovered his passion for architecture and took up his father's unfinished project, determined to complete the house they had always dreamed of. Viva, with her compassionate nature, started a student-run organization focused on promoting kindness and unity in their community.

Their parents watched with pride as the younger generation blossomed under the guidance and inspiration of the stories that had been shared. The Oliver and Smith families continued to hold gatherings, strengthening their bond further with each passing day.

The uncompleted house that had once stood as a symbol of unfinished dreams gradually transformed into a beacon of hope and resilience. Derek poured his heart and soul into completing the project, not just as a tribute to his father but as a testament to the power of friendship and perseverance.

Finally, the day came when the house stood tall, ready to embrace its occupants and the memories yet to be made. The Oliver and Smith families, along with their extended community, gathered to celebrate this milestone. It was a joyous occasion, brimming with laughter, love, and the fulfillment of lifelong dreams.

As they stood on the threshold of the completed house, Cathy, Derek, and Viva knew that their story was just beginning. They had learned the value of friendship, kindness, and the importance of carrying forward the legacies of their fathers. United by a bond that spanned generations, the Oliver and Smith families pledged to continue supporting and uplifting one another. They understood that it was not just bricks and mortar that built a home, but the love, kindness, and shared memories they had cultivated together.

And so, with hearts full of gratitude and determination, they embarked on their journey, knowing that their parents had laid the foundation of love, friendship, and kindness that would guide them through every twist and turn yet to come.

One faithful day, Viva, Cathy, and Derek decided to embark on a delightful adventure to the city zoo. They were excited to witness the beauty and magnificence of various creatures up close. As they entered the zoo, their eyes widened with awe at the sight of elephants gracefully strolling and monkeys swinging from branch to branch. The air filled with the chirping melodies of colorful birds, and the laughter of children echoed through the premises.

Derek, being an avid photographer, was armed with his trusty camera, ready to capture breathtaking shots of the wildlife. His passion for photography knew no bounds, and he sought to reveal the animal kingdom's splendor through the lens of his camera.

Cathy, being an enthusiastic social media enthusiast, couldn't contain her excitement. As Derek clicked away, she eagerly snapped photos with her smartphone, eager to share the zoo's wonders with her online friends. She couldn't wait to post these captivating images on social media platforms, accompanied by witty captions that would surely bring smiles to her followers' faces.

Viva, the ever-curious and compassionate soul, soaked in the sights and sounds of each animal exhibit. She lingered near the lion's habitat, marveling at their majestic manes and powerful presence. She whispered tales of bravery to the regal creatures, as if they could understand her every word.

Moving on, they reached the penguin enclosure, where Viva couldn't help but giggle at their waddling antics. The playful penguins seemed to dance in perfect synchrony, providing endless entertainment for the visitors. Derek captured their joyful frolicking, freezing moments of pure delight in his photographs.

The trio ventured deeper into the zoo, discovering various animal species from all corners of the globe. Cathy, with her keen eye for aesthetics, carefully selected the most captivating moments for her social media posts. From vibrant parrots perched on branches to sleepy koalas lazily cuddling eucalyptus leaves, she sought to share the zoo's enchantment with the world.

As the day drew to a close, they gathered together, reflecting on the memories they had made. Derek proudly displayed his stunning photographs, each one capturing the unique essence of the animals he had encountered. Cathy scrolled through her social media feed, joyfully reading comments from friends and followers who were captivated by her posts.

Viva, ever grateful for the experience, felt a sense of fulfillment. She knew that by appreciating and sharingthe beauty of these incredible creatures, they were shedding light on the importance of conservation and protecting their habitats. Inspired by their day at the zoo, Viva made a vow to become an advocate for animal welfare and raise awareness about the need to safeguard these majestic beings.

With their hearts filled with joy and a deeper appreciation for the wonders of the animal kingdom, the trio bid farewell to the zoo. They knew that the memories they had made and the pictures they had captured would serve as a reminder of the preciousness of all living creatures.

Back at home, Derek spent hours meticulously editing his photographs, bringing out the vibrant colors and intricate details of each animal. He took great care to showcase their grace and beauty, hoping that his images would ignite a sense of wonder and awe in everyone who had the pleasure of viewing them.Cathy, true to her words, continued to share the captivating photographs on her social media accounts. She accompanied each post with educational tidbits about the animals, their natural habitats, and conservation efforts. Her followers were captivated by the striking images and enriched by the knowledge she imparted.

Meanwhile, Viva delved deeper into her research, seeking out opportunities to volunteer at local animal shelters and wildlife conservation organizations. She attended educational workshops and used her platform to spread awareness about the plight of endangered species. Her passion for animals blossomed, fueling her determination to make a difference.

Months passed, and the impact of their zoo visit continued to ripple through their lives. Derek's photographs were showcased in local exhibitions, where people marveled at the wonder captured within each frame. Cathy's social media presence grew, allowing her to connect with like-minded individuals passionate about animal welfare.But most importantly,Viva's dedication to animal advocacy flourished. She embarked on conservation trips to different parts of the

Chapter two

world, contributing to initiatives that protected endangered species and their habitats. Inspired by her journey, she even began writing a book, sharing stories of the animals she encountered and the efforts being made to save them.

On a Friday evening, Derek found himself in the company of a group of energetic and enthusiastic children. he had volunteered to organize an evening full of lively experiences for them, and he couldn't wait to see their faces light up with joy and excitement.

As the children arrived, Derek greeted each one with a warm smile and introduced himself. he had prepared a variety of engaging activities to keep them entertained and make their evening memorable.To kick off the evening, Derek organized an interactive game of charades. The children formed teams, and each team took turns acting out different animals, objects, and actions. Laughter filled the room as they tried to guess the correct answers, their imagination running wild.

Next, Derek set up a mini DIY craft corner. he provided colorful paper, scissors, glue, and various art supplies, allowing the children to let their creativity flow. They made paper airplanes, origami animals, and even personalized friendship bracelets. The room buzzed with excitement as they proudly displayed their creations.

Feeling hungry after all the fun activities, Derek had prepared a small cooking session. he taught the children how to make simple and delicious snacks, like homemade pizzas and fruit skewers. They eagerly followed his instructions, spreading sauce, scattering toppings, and skewering fruits with glee. The aroma of the freshly baked pizzas filled the air, making everyone's mouths water.After the snack break, it was time for some music and dancing. Derek turned on lively, upbeat music, and the children's energy soared. They danced, twirled, and jumped around with wild abandon. Derek joined in the fun, showing off his best dance moves and encouraging the children to let loose and embrace the music.

As the evening came to a close, Derek gathered the children in a circle for a cozy storytelling session. his read their favorite stories aloud, bringing the characters to life and captivating them with his animated storytelling skills. The children eagerly listened, their imaginations whisking them away to magical worlds.

With smiles and laughter, the children bid Derek farewell, grateful for the lively experiences they shared. Derek felt a sense of fulfillment, knowing that he had contributed to creating a memorable and joyful evening for them. he waved goodbye, already looking forward to future opportunities to bring happiness and excitement into their lives once again. Derek went straight to his room, took a shower and start playing video games.

Viva trudged through the front door, exhausted from a long day at school and extra lessons. As she kicked off her shoes and dropped her backpack, her stomach grumbled loudly, reminding her of the empty fridge. She had been looking forward to a satisfying meal to replenish her energy, but to her disappointment, there was nothing to be found. Confused and frustrated, Viva wondered how the fridge had become so bare. She knew her younger brother, Derek, had been home all day, but she never expected him to eat everything. It wasn't like him to be so inconsiderate.

Taking a deep breath, Viva decided to seek out Derek. She found him playing video games in his room, blissfully unaware of her hunger. With a mix of frustration and concern, she gently knocked on his door.
"Derek, can I talk to you for a minute?" Viva asked, trying to keep her tone calm.

Derek turned away from the screen, noticing the exhaustion on Viva's face. "Hey, what's up?" he replied, sensing that something was amiss.

Viva tried to find the right words, not wanting to sound accusatory. "I was really looking forward to a meal when I got home, but the fridge is empty. Did you eat everything?"

Derek's face turned flush with embarrassment. "Yeah, I'm really sorry, Viva. I got carried away with my gaming and lost track of time. I didn't realize you were counting on the food."
Viva could see the sincerity in Derek's eyes, realizing that it was a genuine mistake. She took a moment to collect herself before responding. "It's okay, Derek. I understand that things happen. But next time, please be mindful of others and try not to eat everything without leaving something for everyone else. We're a team, and we need to support each other."
Derek nodded earnestly, feeling remorseful for his thoughtlessness. "You're right, Viva. I should have been more considerate. From now on, I promise to be more mindful and include you in my decisions."
A wave of relief washed over Viva's tired body as she heard Derek's sincere apology. She realized that mistakes happen, even within families, and what truly mattered was their ability to communicate and understand each other's needs.

With hearts now connected and lessons learned, Viva and Derek both went to the kitchen, determined to find a solution to their empty fridge predicament. They decided to work together to come up with a plan that would ensure this wouldn't happen again.
With a smile on her face, Viva proposed, "How about we create a grocery list every week? That way, we can make sure we have enough food for both of us, and we'll take turns going shopping."

Derek nodded eagerly, realizing the importance of taking responsibility and actively participating in the household chores. "That sounds like a great idea, Viva! I'll help with the grocery shopping too."

As they created the grocery list, Viva took into account both of their preferences and dietary needs. She made sure to include healthy options and ingredients they could use to prepare quick and nutritious meals. In the process, they bonded over their shared love for food and discovered new recipes they could try together.

With their conversation wrapped up,she decided to take Matters into her own hands she grabbed her bag,put on her shoes and headed out for the grocery store. Determined to satisfy her snack cravings, she ordered for a pack of Garret Mix popcorn.This famous Chicago popcorn is a blend of Garret's caramel crisp and chees corn popcorn flavors, both made in old fashion copper kettle using secret family recipes,it's her favorite and she felt so happy.

While working home from the store, Viva heard a strange noise from the woods, she was a bit scared because she had never heard anything like that before, the sound was getting louder, she was curious and had to mover closer to the direction of where the sound was coming from. She saw a white and brown kitten yowling and its voice sounded like a long low-pitched moan that usually comes from a cat's throats, that's often drawn-out and quite loud, but the kitten seems to have been attacked by a superior animal and its legs has been injured due to the pressure being placed on the legs, as a result it can't move its legs properly. She quickly carried the kitten away from the woods, and ran home as fast as she can, so she would find a way to take care of the kitten.

As she unloaded the bag into the kitchen counter, she couldn't help but think of what she can do to help the poor kitten. She took the cat to the bathroom, bath it and gave it some first aid-treatment just the way she had been taught in school. She dried the kitten's hair with her hair dryer, bandaged its legs and put the it in her mom's basket.
She was so happy she found a cat, she named the cat Maxy.

Viva was so excited, not knowing how to unveil what she had found at the woods to her brother Derek, she stared at Derek, with smiles on her face, Derek quickly noticed his sister's expressions and was moved to ask what could be the reason behind her happiness.

Viva told her brother everything that had happened when she was coming home, and Derek was eager to see a cat for the first time in his entire existence.
He opened Viva's room and headed straight to the basket where viva had laid Maxy to sleep.

"Oh my goodness! It's real!... Viva, it's a real cat." Derek screamed.

"Yes Derek, it's a real kitten, but it's sick, I wish we had veterinary doctors in town,who can give him a good treatment. Viva said with a sad face. But there are non." she added.

"That's true, how about we take it to the zoo and hand it over to them, what do you think?." He asked.

"No way! That doesn't sound like a good idea, you know cats had been banned from our town, and taking it there would be a huge problem, they might kill Maxy and I don't want to lose Maxy."

"Maxy is just the right name to give this lovely kitty, I wonder how it ended up in the woods, maybe it parents must have traveled from Zamani City because people there really love cats." Derek smile.

"Yes, I think so too, let's keep Maxy." Viva suggested.

"That would be great!, keep it!." The joy on Derek's face has no limit.

They both sat down on the bed, and watched as Maxy sleeps soundly.

It was 6:20pm, Viva, Derek and Maxy were having a good time playing in the house, Maxy seems to be enjoying the moment of being able to play with his new friends. Viva and Derek would run round the table holding a rope while Maxy would chase them in order to get the rope.

Mrs. Smith had just entered the house, but no one noticed until she got closer to them.

"Viva and Derek! What's going on here, what are you guys doing?." She asked.

Viva and Derek paused immediately. "Welcome back Mom." they said at the same time.

"Thanks sweetie, you guys seem distracted, and running round the table like children, are you for real?!." She asked surprisingly.

Viva and Derek were too excited to play with a real cat. They looked at each other and smiled, which got their mom so confused , and curious to ask: "Why are you smiling?, oh I see you really miss childhood play righ?." she asked not expecting any answers as she walked towards the kitchen.

Viva!, Mrs. Smith screamed on the top of her voice. What is this? She yelled from the kitchen, frightened.

Viva and Derek ran to the kitchen, knowing full well the reason for their mom's screams. Derek carried Maxy to his room and shut the door, while Viva was thinking of what to tell her mom because she can see her mom's angry face. When Derek returned to the kitchen, he started to explain.

"Where on earth did you guys see a cat?, I need some explanation Viva." she turned her attention towards Viva being the eldest.

But instead Derek took actions in explaining. "Mom, hurrm….. that's Maxy, Viva found it in the woods, so she decided to bring it home for proper care, it was incredibly injured when Viva saw it, but now It's Better than before, because Viva applied some first-aid treatments so it could get better."

"Proper care? Who is in the rightful position to give a cat proper care viva?."

"The veterinarians." Viva responded.

"Oh!, so you know that, but you decided to bring a cat home?." Her mom asked again.

Viva knew her mom was a disciplinarian, if a good explanation was not given to convince her mom, she would do other wise, probably taking the cat away and hand it over to the police.

"Viva, are you aware that people from this town are not allowed to keep cats?, now listen, I know you really love animals, I can get you a dog, rabbit, rodent, monkey or even a horse, I know you love riding on horses, My dear this cat might put you in danger, and I don't want anything to happen to my children, you know it's just the three of us in this wicked world, so I want you to know that I love you and your brother so much, but that cat!, please take it away."

Tears roll down Viva's face, she loved Maxy and she would do all she can to protect it. "Mom, I know this town forbid cats but I don't know why on earth would anyone hate a cat? I really love Maxy and if I throw him outside, something bad might happen to him. Please mom, just give me some time to think about it, please!"….

Mrs. Smith had never seen her daughter cried because of a pet, so she felt pity for Viva and decided to help her out. "Okay, just make sure you keep it inside always, okay?!. She asked, this time with a smiling face and opened her hands for a hug.

Viva and Derek replied at the same time. Yes we will, they hugged their mom and she kissed them on their cheeks.

"You guys can join me in the kitchen." She said, knowing her children love to help her cook. While cooking they had great conversations and laughter filled the air.

From that day on viva and Derek learned to communicate and respect each other's need when it came to Snacks and pets. Whether it was gaming or enjoying delicious treats,they found a way to strike a balance and share their love for food and fun.

The next day being Saturday, Viva went to visit Cathy, with Maxy on her hands, she had wrapped Maxy like a baby, which made people think she had been holding a baby.
Viva and Cathy were not just best friends; they were like two peas in a pod. Viva had curly brown hair that bounced with every step she took, while Cathy had a head full of golden locks

Chapter three

that shimmered in the sunlight. they shared a special bond. They laughed, played, explored together, and even ride horses together, they behaved like twin sisters, anyone seeing them for the first time will think they were twins, it seemed like they could read each other's thoughts.

Cathy was at the corridor, she had been watching some movies on her laptop. With all seriousness she focused on the interesting movie with out knowing Viva was at her back, Viva tapped her for the first time but she was not aware, Viva tapped her the second time, that was when she turned around.

"Hey Viva, you startled me, what's that on your hands?, who gave you a baby? She asked with curiosity, shifting aside the table in order to get a clear view.

"I knew it!, you thought it was a baby right? But it not."

"What is there then!, tell me."

"I am not telling you, guess!!..." Viva said as she moves backwards.

"Ok! fine, I won't say it a doll because I can't imagine you carrying a doll around, so I would say it probably something you're hiding, so tell me, what are you holding," Cathy asked as she tried to get closer to Viva.

"It's a cat!," Viva revealed.

" Oh my goodness!, is this real? Where did you buy a cat from?." She was flummoxed.

I didn't not buy it, I found it in the woods beside a big tree.

What! Here in Valley town? Cathy muttered.

Yes, I was so surprised when I saw it.

Weren't you scared of it? I mean, I am seeing it for the first time and I can't even touch it. I am scared, but it's so beautiful.

Yes, it is, Com'on touch it, it won't hurt you.

Meow! Maxy cries. It's seeing Cathy for the first time and was frightened.

"See!, you're making him scared ." Viva put Maxy on the floor of the corridor.

"Okay, let me try", Cathy stretches out her hands to touch Maxy, "he seems calm, I like it, Viva did you know it's my first time of touching a cat?,I only see them on movies and my biology Textbook, chapter 56 page 143, I can't forget that page I have always wanted to take pictures with them and now I am holding one with my hands."

"I can take you pictures if you want", viva snapped some pictures on Cathy's phone. "You guys look so cute I still don't know why people from our town don't like cats, they seems harmless to me."

"I agree with you, but I think I would have to find out the reason someday, Viva how do you think people would react if they see Maxy for the first time?." Cathy asked.

"I really don't know what to do, I don't want anyone else to know about Maxy, mom told me to keep it inside but I was just so excited to show you, what should I do?."

"I think you should take good care of it without anybody's knowledge, i wish our town will allow people to train cats again." Cathy suggested

"Me too, if only I can register Maxy like other pets, but I am scared they might hurt him, and I don't want maxy to get hurt."

"No way!, they won't do that, I can tell Dad to register Maxy."

"Wow! Yes that's it a good idea, your Dad won't hurt Maxy, I know. by the way,What's movie are you watching?."

"Jimmy the great Veterinarian; I love how Jimmy treats animals, he is so caring and calm." Cathy explained.

"Wow, I am loving it, the title is perfect, let me get a chair so I can join you." Viva was more than eager to watch the movie. "Cathy, please help me set an alarm on your phone, for 5:30pm." she said as she opened the door to get a chair inside.
Cathy was absent minded, she heard the instructions but didn't acted on it, she was busy caressing Maxy head while watching movies.

"I am back, please pause the movie and explain, so I would be able to understand it."

Cathy paused the movie, and started explaining all she had watched to Viva, Viva understood everything and then they played the movie again as they watched till the end of the movie.

"See!, you're making him scared ." Viva put Maxy on the floor of the corridor.

"Okay, let me try", Cathy stretches out her hands to touch Maxy, "he seems calm, I like it, Viva did you know it's my first time of touching a cat?,I only see them on movies and my biology Textbook, chapter 56 page 143, I can't forget that page I have always wanted to take pictures with them and now I am holding one with my hands."

"I can take you pictures if you want", viva snapped some pictures on Cathy's phone. "You guys look so cute I still don't know why people from our town don't like cats, they seems harmless to me."

"I agree with you, but I think I would have to find out the reason someday, Viva how do you think people would react if they see Maxy for the first time?." Cathy asked.

"I really don't know what to do, I don't want anyone else to know about Maxy, mom told me to keep it inside but I was just so excited to show you, what should I do?."

"I think you should take good care of it without anybody's knowledge, i wish our town will allow people to train cats again." Cathy suggested

"Me too, if only I can register Maxy like other pets, but I am scared they might hurt him, and I don't want maxy to get hurt."

"No way!, they won't do that, I can tell Dad to register Maxy."

"Wow! Yes that's it a good idea, your Dad won't hurt Maxy, I know. by the way,What's movie are you watching?."

"Jimmy the great Veterinarian; I love how Jimmy treats animals, he is so caring and calm." Cathy explained.

"Wow, I am loving it, the title is perfect, let me get a chair so I can join you." Viva was more than eager to watch the movie. "Cathy, please help me set an alarm on your phone, for 5:30pm." she said as she opened the door to get a chair inside.
Cathy was absent minded, she heard the instructions but didn't acted on it, she was busy caressing Maxy head while watching movies.

"I am back, please pause the movie and explain, so I would be able to understand it."

Cathy paused the movie, and started explaining all she had watched to Viva, Viva understood everything and then they played the movie again as they watched till the end of the movie. After watching other movies, the girls went to the pool to swim, Viva and Cathy loved swimming, while swimming, they had nice conversations.

"Viva, I think David is planning to ask me out." Cathy blushed.

"Hmmm, really!, i have always known there was some connections between you two, the way he smiles at you, even holds your hands while walking home, anyone seeing you guys together will know something is going on." Viva chuckles.

"Yea!, I really like David but."….. Cathy paused.

"But what?, what's the problem?." Viva asked.

"Kate told me how much she liked David, but David don't seem to like her at all, I was wondering if I accept his proposal, would that make me a bad person?."

Viva started laughing out loud.

"Why are you laughing?." Cathy asked curiously.

"You might be surprised that David has not even talked to Kate, why are you bothered, if Kate has a crush on David, she should ask him out, she probably would have noticed David's feelings for you, that's why she confined in you at the first place."

"That's true, David feelings for me had been obvious at the very first time we met."

"You can discuss it with David, ask him if he has ever had feelings for Kate, just to know what he has to say, and if he says yes, then tell him to make it clear to Kate that he no longer has any feelings for her."

"What if he says no, what should I do?."

"If he says no, go ahead and accept his proposal."

Cathy's phone started ringing. She got out of the pool to answer the call.

"Viva!, it's David."

Go on answer the phone, and hear what he has to say.

David: Hello, Cathy? It's David. I hope I'm not catching you at a bad time?

Cathy: smiling Hi, David! No, not at all. I was just thinking of you, actually. How are you today?

David: grinning I'm doing great now, especially because I get to talk to you. I have something on my mind that I've been wanting to ask you.

Cathy: curious Oh, really? What is it?.

David: Well, I was wondering if you would do me the honor of going out on a date with me. I've been thinking about it for a while now, and I can't help but feel a special connection between us. I would love the opportunity to get to know you better, Cathy.

Cathy: blushing David, you've truly caught me off guard with that one. I have to say, that connection you mentioned, I've felt it too. Your kindness and genuine nature have been shining through every interaction we've had. I would absolutely love to go on a date with you.

David: grinning ear to ear Really? That's incredible! I couldn't be happier to hear that. I promise you won't regret it, Cathy. I've been planning something special, a date that we'll remember for a long time.

Cathy: excitedly I can't wait to see what you have in mind, David. Knowing you, it's bound to be amazing. I have a feeling this is just the beginning of something wonderful between us.

David: You're right, Cathy. This is only the beginning of our journey. I truly believe that the best is yet to come for us. I have a feeling that our connection will only grow stronger as we continue to explore this path together.

Cathy: softly David, I feel the same way. You've brought so much joy and happiness into my life already. I'm grateful for the bond that's forming between us, and I'm excited to see where it leads.

David: sincerely Thank you for giving me a chance, Cathy. I won't take it for granted. I promise to always cherish and respect you, and to make every moment we share together meaningful and special.

Cathy: can I ask you something?.

David: sure go ahead, ask me anything.

Cathy: do you know Kate browns?.

David: yes, the browns family work for my Dad, I know Kate; but we aren't that close, why do you ask?.

Cathy: Kate says she likes you a lot. So I have been thinking if you guys had feelings before?.

David: oh. no! Cathy, Kate is not really the type of person I like, her characters are all fake, although I don't know much about her but I do know she lies a lot, and live fake life on social media, I don't care.

Cathy: how did you find out about her social media life, I thought I was the only one who knew about it.

David: if she's your friend you can do well to advise her.

Cathy: smiling warmly David, I'll try advice her, well It's my pleasure to have the opportunity to get to know you better. Your thoughtfulness and kindness have already made a significant impact on me, and I can't wait to see where this journey takes us.

David: I'm glad to hear that, Cathy. Your presence in my life is truly a gift, and I can't wait to create unforgettable memories with you. I want to make every moment count, to show you just how much you mean to me.

Cathy: David, you have such a way with words. Your sincerity and genuine affection warm my heart. I feel like I can be completely myself around you, and that's a rare and beautiful thing.

David: You're incredible, Cathy. The more I get to know you, the more I realize just how special you are. Your kindness, intelligence, and the way you light up a room with your smile, it all draws me closer to you. I'm grateful to have you by my side.

Cathy: And I'm grateful to have you by mine, David. It's comforting to know that I have someone like you, someone I can trust and lean on. This connection we're building feels like a once-in-a-lifetime kind of love.

David: It certainly does, Cathy. I believe that when you find someone who brings out the best in you and makes you feel truly alive, you have to hold onto that with everything you have. And that's exactly what I intend to do with you.

Cathy: David, you have my heart, and I promise to give you the love and support you deserve. Our shared journey is just beginning, and I couldn't be more excited for the future we'll create together.

David: Cathy, hearing those words from you fills me with joy and happiness. I promise to be there for you, to support you and love you unconditionally through every twist and turn. Together, we'll build a beautiful and fulfilling life.

Chapter four

Cathy: I can't wait, David. Thank you for choosing me, for seeing something in me that no one else did. I'm grateful for you, for this connection we have, and I can't wait to embark on this incredible adventure with you.

David: The pleasure is all mine, Cathy. You're an extraordinary person, and I'm the luckiest man to have you in my life. Our love story is just beginning, David. And I have a feeling it's going to be filled with laughter, joy, and endless support. With you by my side, I know we can overcome any challenge that comes our way.

David: Absolutely, Cathy. We're a team, and together there's nothing we can't handle. I'll always be there to lift you up, to lend a helping hand, and to celebrate every success with you. You're not alone anymore; we're in this together.

Cathy: That means the world to me, David. Knowing that I have someone as kind, caring, and reliable as you in my corner gives me strength and reassurance. Thank you for being the incredible person you are.

David: Thank you, Cathy, for accepting me and for seeing the best in me. It's truly an honor to be the person by your side, supporting and loving you. We're going to make a great team, and I can't wait to see what the future holds for us.

Cathy: Likewise, David. The future is bright, and I have no doubt that it will be filled with incredible moments and boundless love. Let's make the most of every day, cherishing and nurturing our connection, and making beautiful memories together.

David: Agreed, Cathy. Let's seize this opportunity to create a love story that will inspire others and bring happiness to both of us. Having you in my life is a blessing, and I'm excited to see how our journey unfolds.

Cathy: As am I, David. Together, we'll navigate through life's ups and downs, supporting each other every step of the way. With our love and friendship, anything is possible. Thank you for being the amazing person you are and for brightening my world.

David: Thank you for being the same, Cathy. You bring so much light into my life, and I'm grateful for every moment we share. Here's to the beginning of our beautiful love story and the beautiful future that awaits us, will be free tomorrow evening?.

Cathy: of course I am free, what are your plans?.

David: I want to surprise you, so by 4:30 tomorrow, I will come pick you up.

Cathy: wow, I love surprises, I can't wait to see you tomorrow.

David: you too, can't wait to see your beautiful face.

Cathy: Awwn! That's so sweet.

David: what are you doing now?.

Cathy: swimming with Viva.

David: oh Viva is there with you, send my regards to her, she must have been waiting for you all along.

Cathy: don't worry about her, she's definitely doesn't have a problem with that.

David: let me allow you enjoy your swimming with Viva, I will call back later at night.
Cathy: okay, I will be expecting your calls.

David: sure!, take good care of yourself.

Cathy: I will, and you too.

David: bye.

Cathy: bye.

The Call ended, as Cathy walked up to Viva.

Coughing….."oh am coughing, Arhhhh .

"Stop it Viva, I know that's a fake cough."

"I never knew my friend could be so in love with someone. Cathy, you spent almost two hours speaking with your lover."

"Com'on Viva!, it's not up to two hours."

"How would you know, when you 're busy expressing your feelings to David

Wait a minute!, did you overheard our conversation?.

Of course I did, even though you speaking with a low voice, I heard everything, I never knew you had been madly in love with David.

Of course, I am so in love with him and I am more than excited to go out with him on Sunday evening.

Tomorrow?.

Yes, but I really don't know the dress to wear, will you help me out?.

Sure, let's go check out some of your new clothes, maybe you'll find something nice to wear from it.

We went to Cathy's room, her wardrobe was filled with beautiful clothes. As they proceeded in searching for better outfit, Viva finally saw a very beautiful black dress.

Cathy look! This dress is so beautiful.

Oh my little black dress, I think you're right, I have a lace up heel and a clutch bag.

Perfect! Now you're set for a cute and classy date night.

Awwwn! What will I do without you Viva, you're such a sweetheart, come give me a hug.

They hugged each other and indulged themselves together in a very good conversation.

Maxy's meow distracted them, as he walked up to Viva.

Oh my sweet little Maxy is awake, it seems he is hungry, Cathy what do you have for Maxy?.

There's milk and cheese in the refrigerator and some fried chicken thighs.

Maxy drank some milk and ate the fried chicken but refused to eat the cheese because he was satisfied.

"Viva it's 6:15pm already Cathy said".

'Oh no! I told mom I would be back by 6:00pm, Mr Tomas would be joining us for dinner'.

Hey, I am so sorry, I totally forgot you told me to set an alarm for 5:30".

"Yea I really have to go now", Viva said as she turn around put on her shoes.

Cathy was about to call her mom, 'Can I call my mom to come pick you up"?.

"No! You don't have to do that, I'll just take a Uber instead"

While they were still talking, the honk of a car distracted them.

"Oh my mom is here! Good for you Viva, she'll take you home" Cathy said with a smile.

"Good evening ladies!!, how are you guys doing? Cathy mom said as she hugged them, Viva dear weren't you Suppose to be at home by this time, you'll be late for dinner".
At this point the two girls were more than surprised, they gave each other a quick look, trying to figure out how in the world she knew about the dinner.

"You guys looked surprised, oh Viva!, your mom invited me but I wasn't sure because of my business trip, so i declined.

Oh that's true! So who is the guest? Cathy asked.

It's Mr Tomas, Mom's friend, they kinda like each other, but I am still getting to know him, here!, we took some pictures together last week at the park. She showed some pictures of Mr. Tomas on her phone.

"Wow he looks cute", Cathy complimented.

"Oh I know him, Mrs. Oliver said.

"How did you get to know him?." Cathy asked.

"Mr. Tomas had been my bank manager for three years now, Cathy, your Dad knows him too".

"Bank manager!"?, the two girls asked with surprise.

"Yes, is there any problem with that ?" Mrs. Oliver asked not knowing why the girls were surprised about the news.

"Mom, Mr. Tomas told Cathy's mom that he owned Tombass Company, he even mentioned that he will employ Derek during holidays period in order to help him save some money before school resumes".

"Tombass Company is one of the biggest companies in town,why would he say something like that, I have known Tomas for three years now as a banker, so I have no idea if he says he owns Tombass Company, maybe it's his family Company or what do you think?".

"I think I have to find out the truth and the only way to know is to browse it online, Viva brought out her phone from her bag, searching on Google, oh my goodness! Cathy look what I found!",She said while scrolling up and down of her phone.

"What's that Viva, What did you find out?" Cathy said anxiously,while she moved closer to Viva with all eagerness to see what Viva was about to show her.

"My dear you can read it out so we can listen!" Mrs. Oliver was so curious to know what Goggle search has to say about Tombass Company.

"Okay Ma, I read :"Tombass Company is a retail store chain that offers many wholesale or retail goods for lower prices. This Company has over 2 million global workers. As one of the world's largest public cooperation,Tombass is a family-owned business controlled by the Tomsons family. Tombass's goal is to provide fair and low prices on consumer goods.it's Headquarters are located at bugulie center, Tombass is owned by its shareholders. The Tomsons family is the largest shareholder of Tombass holding 50% of the company's shares. The Tomsons family acquired such high ownership of the company because they are the descendants of Luke Tomson who founded the company"....

"Hold on Viva! I don't understand, are you trying to say Mr Tomas is related to Luke Tomson? What is Mr . Tomas last name"? Cathy said with a confused expression.

"I am also as confused as you are...ok let's find out!".

"Viva!, Just type (who are Luke Tomson's descendants?) on your browser, then enter the company's website, I think you'll find all the details or informations you need on their website. do it let's see what you'll find".

"Okay, let's do this!" Viva said as she started searching. Oh here's something interesting, I read again: Luke Tomson has three sons Richard, Bill and William, and ten grandchildren Samuel, Daniel, Benita, Justine,Michael, Sandra, Mary, Bob, Racheal,and Rose, he also has three great grandchildren, khole and Anderson and Scott.

Chapter five

They all stared at each other, without knowing what to say…. Mrs. Oliver decided to break the silence, Com'on girls, I can give you a ride you want to. She said trying to ease the tension.

"That's a good idea" they replied together.

Mrs. Oliver went to the Garage where she had packed her car, she quickly hopped in her car and took the girls while she drove off.

Mrs. Smith had invited Mr. Tomas over for dinner, and they were enjoying a lovely evening at her welcoming home. Derek, sat at the table as well, adding to the lively atmosphere.

Mr. Tomas couldn't help but feel his heart fluttering, as he had always had a mysterious plan on the Smith's Family, so he tried flirting with Mrs. Smith in order to Execute his plans.

Mrs. Smith knew Viva was supposed be at home with them but she didn't worry because she knew Viva won't miss having dinner with them.
As they chatted and savored the delicious meal prepared by Mrs. Smith, laughter filled the air. The conversation flowed effortlessly, everyone enjoying each other's company.

"Mrs. Smith, you're a great cook, I had never had such a delicious meal for ages. I wish I have some like you to call my own, don't worry very soon we will visit Asia countries for a vacation just me, you and my lovely kids Derek and Viva!. I know Derek and Viva must have been enjoying good meals all the time".he complimented her.

Mrs. Smith knew she was a good cook since she learnt very well from her mother, she just smiled back at Mr. Tomson, thanks so much Mr. Tomas.

"Com'on you can just call me Tomas instead", he said with a huge smile on his face as he stood up and head towards the corridor, Excuse me please I have to answer a Business call, the company has been disturbing me much this days.

Mr. Tomas spent quite some time receiving calls before he joined them again and start another conversation.
My dear, I just wish i could take you out on a shopping at Dubai so you can get yourself some very expensive jewels and clothes because I just received an wedding invitation from my friend from Germany, he is getting married next month and I want you and I to be there, please don't

say know because I will be the happiest man on earth if you agree, while he was yet speaking....

The front door swung open, and in walked Viva, Cathy, and Mrs. Oliver, Everyone paused for a while,Mrs. Smith had been expecting her lovely daughter, the smiles on her face lit up with love when she saw Viva.

Mrs. Smith welcomed them with hugs, Mrs. Oliver, you made it, I felt bad when you told me you wouldn't be able to come around, how was your business trip? Mrs.smith asked with a smile.

"Everything's doing great thanks, and you?." Mrs.Oliver replied.

"Same here, oh! Over here, come let me introduce you to someone".she took Mrs Smith by the hand to the dining.

Cathy And Viva had already sat down beside Derek and waiting for their moms to come.

Mr. Tomas was so shocked when he saw Mrs. Oliver, his heart started beating fast,he wasn't really expecting her to be there. he murmured to himself," am a mess right now, what will I do? Should I act like I don't know her? while he was still in deep thoughts, Mrs. Smith interrupted him.

"Hey, meet Mrs. Oliver, and Mrs. Oliver meet Mr. Tomas, the both of them greeted each other with smiles, as they all reclined on the table to enjoy the meal, they engaged their selves in a conversation.

So Mr. Tomas, how are you enjoying the food? Viva asked wearing a fake smile.

Oh dear your mom is the best cook,I can't say less, he replied fast as if he had been expecting the question.
He tried to crack some jokes which made them laugh, for a while, he felt relaxed and completely forgot about everything.Meanwhile Mrs. Oliver had been looking for the right time to ask her questions,and she told her self "it is now".

Mr. Tomas, how is work going? Asked Mrs. Oliver

Mr.Tomas started shaking in fear, he tried so hard to hide his feelings but to no Avail,Everyone noticed how uncomfortable he is feeling,Derek and his mom were in great shock.

Mrs. Oliver proceeded with her questions, assuming Mr. Tomas didn't hear her first question. so Mr. Tomas, how is Mr. Dean your work assistant?

This time Mr.Tomas managed to respond, Oh my P A is doing just fine, how is your work going too? He asked in return but before Mrs. Oliver reply, Mrs. Smith interrupted the conversation.

"Tomas, you've never told me you have a personal Assistant named Mr. Dean, you and Mrs. Oliver seem to know each other well." Mrs. Smith was curious.

Mr. Tomas faked a smile and tried lying. Mrs. Smith you see, Our company is so big and we employ a lot of workers almost every three months, Mr. Dean is more like a Brother to me. he said hoping Mrs. Oliver won't notice anything in his reply to Mrs.Smith.

"But you and Mr. Dean don't seem to act like friends instead you act like enemies." Mrs.Oliver added.

"Mrs. Oliver, Mr.Dean is my assistant and I don't have any issues with him."

Viva had been quiet all through, thinking of how she can add to the conversation without any disrespect,so she came up with a plan. She coughed a little as if clearing her throat in order to speak clearly before asking her questions, hmmm! Mr. Tomas, hope you're enjoying your dinner?.

'Oh my dear, yes I am really enjoying it'. this time he replied with confidence thinking he had gain every one trust.

"I see, so where do you work"?. Viva asked again.

Not knowing what to say, he started acting like someone choking from food.

Oh Mr. Tomas you can drink some water, Viva said while stretching her hands for a glass of water.here you go! She handed him a glass of water.

Oh thank you my dear, you're such a good kid,and your mom would be so proud of you. He said, trying to change the topic.

Thank you, Mr. Tomas, so I ask again, where do you work? Viva asked and Cathy supported: yes Mr. Tomas, I am also curious about your work because I would like to work with you.

Mr. Tomas felt a sharp pain in his brain due to stress, he knew that was a bad sign, every one is getting curious, what should I do? He asked himself,and finally decided to say something. Huummm, I, I, I, own a company named Tombass. It's a very popular company with a lot of customers, you see I am a very gentle and wealthy man, Cathy you said you would like to work with me, oh you are welcome to join us in making our company grow.

Mr. Tomas can I see your Identification card?,because I am more than Excited. Cathy asked.

Sure! Sure! Here it is, he brought out his Identification Card and gave it to Cathy. Cathy glanced at the card and passed it to her mom while Mrs. Oliver pass it lastly to Viva and Viva looked at it for something and started reading out what is written on the card both the Name, Age, Address.

Immediately she was done reading, Viva, Mrs. Oliver, and Cathy stared at each other and started laughing out loud at once. Everyone was so surprised, including Mr. Tomas, he felt very Embarrassed.

Viva, is there something am missing? Derek asked because he noticed his sister's unusual character.

Derek! Yes, you and mom are missing a lot, Mr. Tomas here had been lying to you and mom for a long time, mom!, Mr. Tomas said that he own a house at Midway close, he has three cars, he is from France, he own Tombass company and he is single, Mom!, it's all lies, Tombass Company is Owned by Luke Tomson and Mr Tomas is not anywhere found in the names of Luke Tomson's descendants, I also overheard him talking to someone on the phone, telling the person that he is about to execute his deep plans and the name here in his Identification Card is Tomas Quinn not anywhere near the Tomson's Family, he has a wife named Elizabeth and twins children, Alex and Alexis, he is from Texas and he work at bundie Bank. Mr. Tomas what other lies have you told my mom?.

Mr. Tomas was speechless and he had never in his life been this embarrassed, he quickly knelt down before Mrs. Smith and started confessing.
Mrs. Smith I am so so so sorry for everything I never knew it would end this way, please forgive me!.. I was hired by Mr. khan to get your late husband's documents and make you sign it, I thought flirting with you would make it fast but I wasn't thinking well, please forgive me….

What's Going on here! So you mean you were hired? And what documents are you talking about? What are you supposed to do with the documents? Derek asked what angers in his eyes.

Before you Dad die he sign a contract of $600,000,000 which was supposed to be deposited into his account on the 1st of July with the additional amount of $200,000, 000 from the real estate team. Mr. Khan was aware of the contract and decided to have the money for himself he has tried threatening your Dad to give him half of the money but your Dad refuses which ended in death. I believe Mr. Khan killed your dad, and as your dad's account officer, he threatened to kill me and my family if I did not find a way for your mom to sign the papers, it's only your mom that can sign it, he threatened never to tell your mom about the money. I am so sorry, I don't want to lose my job and my family. He started crying.

But why didn't you involve the police to arrest him? Derek asked again.

The police? No way! Don't do that , Mr Khan has Badboys all over the country, even the police can't stop him. But I have all our calls recorded on my computer.

There was a knock on the door and everyone stood up at once alarmed. Who is there?, Viva asked as she moved closer to the door, but there was no response, she asked again, who is there? this time with a more louder voice, Mr. Tomas hid himself behind Derek, shivering so bad as if someone poured him a very cold water. Viva took courage to open the door, it was Cathy's Dad he was on headphones.

"Oh Mr. Oliver, it's you! Good Evening sir." Viva said with Great relief.

"Viva! How are you doing?, Is my wife and daughter here?." He asked.

"Yes! Yes, come in." Viva opened the door wide for Mr. Oliver to enter.

Everyone was relieved at once when they finally saw Mr. Oliver.
Dad! Cathy ran to hug her father, her mother joined them.

"My Angel, how are you doing? Sweetie, how are you." He asked his wife and daughter with smiles on his face.

"we are fine dad, we thought it was someone else's on the door."

"Oh no you guys must have been expecting a visitor, Hello everyone, Good Evening Mrs. Smith, Mr. Tomas, and Derek."

"Good evening Mr. Oliver welcome." they replied, except From Mrs. Smith, she had been in deep thought without taking notice of anything around her, immediately viva realizes that her mother was in deep thought, she quickly touched her mom to make sure she doesn't get high blood pressure again.

"Mom! Hey, stop thinking everything is going to be fine." I promise you.

"Mrs. Smith, are you okay?." Mr. Oliver asked, showing concern.

Mrs. Oliver told her husband everything that has happened and he was very surprised.
Mr. Oliver was a deputy general, when he heard everything he assured Mrs. Oliver that he and his crews would do some investigating on the matter and invite Mr. Tomas to come to the police station for more investigations, he asked for the Documents.

Derek searched his late father's room for the documents and found it inside his office locker, he brought them out and handed it over to Mr. Oliver.

"Mrs. Smith I will bring your husband's lawyer so you can sign the documents and transfer the money to your account." Mr. Oliver assured Mrs. Smith as he put the documents inside his bag And call for a backup crew to escort Mr. Tomas to the police department.

Chapter six

"Dad please do all you can to make sure you arrest Mr. Khan." Cathy pleaded.

"It's okay my dear everything will be okay, we just have to do more investigations and find more evidence, and we will be needing Mr. Tomas."

The car siren sounds became louder as it approached the house, Mr. Oliver stood up after going through the Documents. The police officers knocked on the door, Mr. Oliver opened the door and talked to the officers for some minutes then returned inside.

"Mrs. Smith, we will be leaving some officers to assist you, let me introduce you to officers Ben, Gadro, Jude and Raphael. Jude will be monitoring the front, Gadro the right, Ben the left and Raphael the back, take this if you notice anything unusual press this alarm button to keep everyone alert and call me immediately, is that okay Mrs. Smith?, do you have any questions?."

"No, thank you so much Mr. Oliver, I really appreciate your support, I totally understand and I just have one question to ask."

"go ahead, ask your questions."

"What will happen to Mr. Khan when you eventually catch him?."

"He will be punished by the law, don't worry I will make sure he never goes free. by 10:30am in the morning we will also need you at the police department for some important information and please do well to tell the police all you know about the matter."

"No problem Mr. Oliver, I will do just that". Mrs Smith replied with a satisfied smile.

The police took Mr. Tomas away and Mr and Mrs. Oliver and their daughter Cathy, followed them. In the house was Mrs. Smith and her children, and the police officers who were guarding them.

Derek was finding it hard to sleep, he quietly walked into Viva's bedroom, he sat on the bedside. "Hey Viva, are you sleeping already?".

"Derek, I just can't sleep after everything that has happened". Viva said with a very low voice.

"I admire you a lot. Where did you get that information from? I mean everything you said about Mr. Tomas?" He asked curiously.

Viva held his hands, "have I ever told you about Darlington?."

"No you haven't, who is Darlington?" He asked.

"I met Darlington at school after extra lessons. He helped me with my Assignments, which I had to do a lot of research on, but Darlington made it very easy for me to understand. He used his computer and it seems he is a hacker too."

"A hacker? Wow! So you mean after your Assignments you told him about Mr. Tomas?."

"No no way! This evening at Cathy's house, Mrs. Oliver exposed Mr. Tomas work as a banker instead of a company owner, i had to browse every detail about Mr. Tomas but i found nothing, so i called Jason to help me out, he asked for his name, surname and picture and as after just 5 minutes, he sent me every details I needed, I was very surprised when I saw the whole information and my heart broke into pieces, but I had to put my self together in order to stop any further damages being made, I really don't know how mom would be feeling by now, even though she is a strong woman."

"Hmmm!, I am the man here but I can't seem to make a difference, I am just helpless, what can I do to help? What's your next plan?." He asked in a sad voice.

"My lovely brother, you are the best thing that has ever happened to this family, you are not weak, you are a very strong person with big heart, now listen to me, all I want you to do is to take good care of yourself and mom, tomorrow by God's grace, we will stick together and make sure we do everything to get back what is ours. but I want you to sleep, so you'll get your self some energy."

"Thanks so much viva, can I sleep in your room please?."

"Sure! You can sleep here, let's pray so you can turn off the lights."

"They kneel down to pray together, after which they turn off the light and sleep off."

It's 7:30 in the morning, Mrs. Smith has invited the police officers to have breakfast with them, at first they rejected the offer but she kept insisting, so they joined them in the dining room to eat. Mrs. Smith was making sure that everything that happened would not disturb her children in anyways.

"Viva, pass me the pancakes." Mrs. Smith ordered.

Mrs. Smith took the pancakes from Viva and passed it to Gadro, one of the officers. She also started a conversation.

"So Ben, tell us something about yourself, like your favorite food, colors or place."

Ben cleared his throat. "I guess my favorite food is Avocado toast, chicken and waffles. I also like going to the beachside for a clearer view of the beach beauty and lastly I don't think I have a favorite color, I love all colors."

The room was filled with laughter as they enjoyed their breakfast.

Mrs. Smith, accompanied by her children Viva and Derek, made their way to the police headquarters, determined to uncover the truth about her husband's death and the deceitful actions of Mr. Tomas. Relieved to find him still in custody, they were determined to get the answers they needed.

As they sat down in the interrogation room, Mrs. Smith took a deep breath and looked into Mr. Tomas' eyes. "Why did you pretend to be the owner of Tombass Company when you're actually a banker?" she asked, her voice filled with a mix of anger and desperation.

Mr. Tomas avoided direct eye contact, shifting uncomfortably in his seat. "I... I needed money," he mumbled. "I thought if I could convince you to sign those documents, I could access your husband's wealth and solve my financial problems."

Viva, who had been silently observing, jumped in. "And what about Mr. Khan? Why was he so determined to make Mrs. Smith sign those documents?"

Mr. Tomas hesitated, realizing he was digging himself into a deeper hole. "I... I'm not sure," he stammered, sweat forming on his forehead. "Mr. Khan, he threatened me. He said he had connections and would ruin my life if I didn't comply."

Derek, always the calm and analytical one, leaned forward. "We need to delve deeper into this, Mr. Tomas. It seems there are more layers to this story than meets the eye. We want justice for our family."

At that moment, Detective Oliver entered the room. He had promised to conduct further investigations on Mr. Khan and was ready to share his findings with the group.

"Mrs. Smith, Viva, Derek, I've gathered some valuable information," Detective Oliver began. "Mr. Khan has a reputation for shady dealings, and it appears he targeted your late husband as a potential victim. His signature on the documents would have granted him access to a significant amount of wealth."

Mrs. Smith's eyes widened, realizing the gravity of the situation. "We must stop him," she said determinedly. "We can't let him get away with this."

Detective Oliver nodded in agreement. "I assure you, Mrs. Smith, we won't rest until we have enough evidence to bring Mr. Khan to justice. We'll also ensure that Mr. Tomas faces the consequences of his actions."

With renewed hope and determination, Mrs. Smith, Viva, Derek, and Detective Oliver formed a plan to expose Mr. Khan's deceitful intentions and bring him to justice. They gathered any evidence they could find, preparing a strong case against him.

Meanwhile, Detective Oliver reached out to his network of contacts, digging deeper into Mr. Khan's past. He discovered a pattern of fraudulent activities and illegal schemes that Mr. Khan had conducted throughout the years. Armed with this information, they knew they had to act swiftly to protect Mrs. Smith and ensure justice was served.

At the same time, Mrs. Smith received anonymous tips and messages, warning her of potential dangers and urging her to stay vigilant. Despite the fear and uncertainty, she refused to let fear consume her. With the support of her friend Mrs. Oliver and the determination to seek justice for her late husband, she pressed on.

One day, as they gathered to review the progress of their investigation, a breakthrough occurred. Detective Oliver had uncovered a hidden link between Mr. Khan and an international money laundering operation. It seemed that Mr. Khan had been using his connections to exploit vulnerable individuals and funnel money through various illegal channels.

With this evidence in hand, they approached the authorities, presenting a compelling case against Mr. Khan. The investigation gained momentum, and soon the truth about Mr. Khan's illicit activities came to light. His web of lies unraveled, leaving no room for escape.

In a dramatic turn of events, Mr. Khan was apprehended, and the pieces of the puzzle started falling into place. Mrs. Smith finally felt a sense of relief as she saw justice being served. She knew her late husband's memory was being honored, and his legacy protected.

As the legal proceedings continued, Mrs. Smith, Viva, and Derek supported one another through the emotional toll the events had taken. Though the journey had been arduous, their friendship had grown stronger in the face of adversity.

Months later, the trial against Mr. Khan concluded, and he was found guilty of multiple charges, including fraud, forgery, and conspiracy. The sense of closure brought solace to Mrs. Smith and allowed her to start the process of healing.

With the support of her family and the knowledge that justice had prevailed, Mrs. Smith was able to move forward, determined to rebuild her life and honor her late husband's memory. She knew that he would be proud of her strength and perseverance.

And as time passed, Mrs. Smith became a symbol of resilience for others who had experienced similar injustices. She used her experience and newfound knowledge to advocate for stricter regulations and protections against fraud and deception, aiming to prevent others from falling prey to individuals like Mr. Khan.

Days turned into weeks, Mrs. Smith and her children continued to support each other on their respective journeys. Viva diligently studied for her exams.
after a long day at school, Viva returned home feeling famished. Her stomach growled loudly, reminding her that she hadn't eaten since lunchtime. Eagerly, she opened the front door, expecting the comforting aroma of home-cooked food to welcome her.

Her heart sank as she stepped into an empty kitchen. The cupboards were bare, and the fridge offered nothing but a lonely carton of milk. Disappointment etched across her face as she realized that Derek had devoured all the food in the house, likely along with his friends.

Overwhelmed by hunger, frustration, and exhaustion, Viva's eyes welled up with tears. She had been looking forward to a nourishing meal, a moment of solace after a challenging day. She could sense her dreams of becoming a veterinarian slipping away, overshadowed by the weight of disappointment.
As Viva headed out to grab some food, she felt a familiar sense of excitement bubbling inside her. The sun was shining, casting a warm glow over the streets, and Viva couldn't help but let her mind wander to her dream of becoming a veterinarian. The idea of helping animals in need and making a difference in their lives fueled her determination every day.

As she walked towards her favorite cafe, Viva spotted her friend Cathy standing by a nearby park. Cathy, a compassionate and caring soul, shared Viva's love for animals. They had bonded over their shared passion ever since they were kids.

"Hey Viva!" Cathy called out, a bright smile lighting up her face. "What brings you here?"

"I was just heading to grab some food," Viva replied, joining Cathy by the park's entrance. "But I can never pass up the chance for some good company. What about you?"

Cathy's eyes sparkled with excitement. "Well, you won't believe what happened today. I came across a stray dog in the park, and it looked like it had injured its paw."

Viva's face lit up. "Oh wow! Did you help it?"

Chapter seven

Cathy nodded. "I did my best to calm it down and bandage its paw. But I think it needs more extensive care than I can provide. That's where you come in, my aspiring veterinarian! I thought you might have some ideas."

Viva couldn't hide her enthusiasm, her heart skipping a beat at the opportunity to help an animal in need. "Of course, Cathy! Let's head over to the park and see if we can find the dog. Maybe I can take a look at its injury and provide some immediate care."

Together, Viva and Cathy strolled to the park, fueled by their shared passion for helping animals. As they arrived, a gentle, scruffy-looking dog sat on the grass, whimpering softly. Its injured paw was clearly visible, making Viva's heart ache.

Approaching the dog slowly, Viva knelt down with a soothing tone in her voice. After gaining its trust, she carefully examined the injury and concluded that it needed immediate attention from a veterinarian. But she didn't stop there.

Viva and Cathy decided to take the dog to a nearby animal shelter. They explained the situation to the compassionate staff, who agreed to provide the necessary care and find the dog a loving forever home.

Over the next few weeks, Viva's commitment to becoming a veterinarian grew stronger. She discussed her experiences with the injured dog in the park with her parents, who were impressed with her compassion and determination.

Her Mother Mrs. Smith, had always been supportive of her dreams. She sat down with her one evening, wanting to learn more about her aspirations.

"Viva, I am really proud of you," Mrs. Smith said, a warm smile on her face. "Your passion for helping animals is truly inspiring. But have you thought about the challenges that come with pursuing a career as a veterinarian?"

Viva nodded, her conviction evident. "Yes, Mom, I have. I know it won't be easy, but I believe that if I truly love what I do, I'll find a way to overcome any obstacles. I want to make a difference in the lives of animals and contribute to their well-being."

Derek chimed in, his voice filled with pride. "We believe in you, Viva. We've seen your dedication and kindness towards animals all these years. And if anyone can make a difference, it's you."

Feeling encouraged by her Mom and Derek unwavering support, Viva shared the whole story with Darlington during their weekly holiday. Darlington, with his wealth of knowledge and life experiences, listened intently.

After Viva shared her aspirations and her encounter with the injured dog, Darlington leaned back in his chair and gave her a thoughtful smile. "Viva, always remember that following your passion is a key to living a fulfilling life. You have the heart and the drive to make a real impact. But it's important to equip yourself with knowledge and experience along the way."

He continued, "Why don't you look for opportunities to volunteer at local veterinary clinics or animal shelters? It will give you hands-on experience, help you build connections and solidify your understanding of the field."

Viva's eyes sparkled with excitement as she realized the possibilities. "Darlington, that's a brilliant idea! I'm going to start searching for volunteering opportunities right away. Thank you for your guidance."

With her Mom, Derek and Darlington's encouragement, Viva felt more determined than ever to pursue her dream of becoming a veterinarian. She knew that the road ahead would be challenging, but their support fueled her passion and gave her the strength to overcome any obstacles that lay in her path.

Armed with her newfound inspiration, Viva wasted no time in beginning her search for volunteer positions. She reached out to new local veterinary clinics and animal shelters, expressing her eagerness to lend a hand.

One snow-filled morning, Viva received a call from the Sunny Paws Animal Clinic. They were thrilled to have her join their team as a volunteer. Overjoyed, she eagerly accepted the opportunity and couldn't wait to contribute to the well-being of the animals in their care.

At the clinic, Viva was welcomed with open arms by the staff. Dr. Matthew, the lead veterinarian, took her under her wing and showed her the ropes. Viva quickly learned how to assist during examinations, prepare medication, and care for the animals in the recovery area. She observed surgeries and even had the chance to help during simple procedures.

Her kindness and dedication soon became evident to both the staff and the furry patients. Viva's gentle touch and soothing words provided comfort to even the most anxious animals. She made it a point to spend time with each patient, showering them with love and attention.

Word of Viva's compassion spread throughout the clinic, and people started requesting her assistance specifically. It wasn't long before Viva became a beloved presence in the lives of the animals and their owners.

Through her experiences at Sunny Paws Animal Clinic, Viva learned valuable lessons about animal care and the challenges veterinarians face. She had the opportunity to witness both the joys and heartbreaks of the profession. Despite the challenges, her determination remained unwavering, only intensified by her newfound knowledge.

After spending several months volunteering, Viva noticed the positive impact her presence had on the animals and their owners. She understood that her genuine care and empathy played a significant role in their healing process. It was during this time that she realized she had the ability not only to heal animals physically but also to provide emotional support to their humans.

With this profound realization, Viva set her sights on becoming a veterinarian who focused not only on medical expertise but also on creating a warm and comforting environment for pets and their families. She wanted to build a place where every animal would feel safe, loved, and understood.

With each passing day, Viva's dream of becoming a veterinarian burned brighter. She was also part of the most intelligent students who were given scholarships to study in Netford University, she can't wait to start a new journey. her unfaltering spirit and genuine kindness endeared her to those around her. The road ahead might be challenging, but Viva, with her unwavering determination and compassionate heart, was eager to learn and grow. One day, after class, Viva approached her Biology teacher, Ms. Johnson, to discuss her passion for animal welfare.

"Ms. Johnson, I've been volunteering at a veterinary clinic, and it has really ignited my desire to make a difference in the lives of animals. I was wondering if you had any suggestions on how I can further educate myself on this topic," Viva said, her eyes filled with excitement.
Ms. Johnson smiled warmly and replied, "I'm thrilled to see your passion, Viva. Animal welfare is indeed a noble cause. There are several ways you can expand your knowledge. Firstly, I recommend enrolling in courses or workshops that focus on veterinary medicine or animal behavior. This will give you a deeper understanding of their physical and mental needs."

Viva nodded eagerly, taking notes of Ms. Johnson's advice. "That sounds fantastic, Ms. Johnson! Are there any particular courses or workshops you'd recommend?"
Ms. Johnson pondered for a moment before responding. "Well, there's a local animal shelter that occasionally organizes educational workshops on animal behavior and care. They invite professionals from different fields to speak and share their expertise. It's a great opportunity to learn and network with like-minded individuals. I'll give you their contact information. I'm sure they would be thrilled to have someone as passionate as you attending."

Overjoyed by the suggestion, Viva thanked Ms. Johnson profusely. She couldn't wait to explore this new avenue of learning and make connections with others who shared her love for animals. The following week, Viva attended her first workshop at the animal shelter. As she mingled with other attendees and listened to the passionate speakers, Viva felt a sense of belonging. She engaged in thought-provoking discussions, shared her experiences, and absorbed as much knowledge as she could.

Inspired by the workshop, Viva decided to take her newfound insight and share it with her fellow students. She organized a small gathering where she presented what she had learned about animal behavior, welfare, and the importance of responsible pet ownership.

Her classmates were captivated by Viva's enthusiasm and the depth of her knowledge. They asked questions, shared their own experiences, and brainstormed ways they could contribute to animal welfare. Viva, with her kind and patient nature, guided them through the discussions, encouraging empathy and understanding.

From that day forward, Viva's classmates saw her as the go-to person for any animal-related questions or concerns. Her kind and helpful nature extended beyond the classroom, even reaching her own neighbors.

One evening, as Viva was watering her plants in the front yard, her neighbor Mr. Harrison approached her with a puzzled expression. "Hello, Viva! I've noticed you're quite knowledgeable about animals. I recently adopted a rescue dog, and I could use some advice on how to make her feel more at ease in her new home. Do you have any suggestions?"

Viva smiled warmly and put her watering can aside. "Of course, Mr. Harrison! I'd be happy to help. Firstly, congratulations on adopting a rescue dog. They truly have a special place in our hearts. One important thing to keep in mind is to give your new furry friend some time to adjust. Shelter dogs have often experienced trauma or abandonment, so they may feel anxious or fearful initially. Creating a safe and comfortable environment is key."

Viva went on to explain the importance of establishing a routine, providing plenty of mental and physical stimulation, as well as offering a cozy space for the dog to retreat to when they need some alone time. She also emphasized the significance of positive reinforcement training techniques and the benefits of patience and consistency in building trust.

Mr. Harrison listened attentively, taking notes on his phone. "Thank you so much, Viva! I really appreciate your guidance. I want my new companion to feel loved and secure in her new home."

Viva nodded, her eyes glowing with warmth. "You're very welcome, Mr. Harrison. If you have any more questions or need further help along the way, don't hesitate to reach out. I'm here to assist you in any way I can."

Word of Viva's knowledge and willingness to help quickly spread among her neighbors. They admired her passion and sought her advice on various topics, such as pet nutrition, managing behavioral issues, and even creating wildlife-friendly gardens. Viva never turned anyone away, always taking the time to listen, empathize, and offer her insights.

Through her conversations with her neighbors, Viva not only educated them about animals but also inspired them to become more responsible and compassionate pet owners. The community began to bloom with a stronger awareness of animal welfare and a shared commitment to making a positive impact.

As Viva continued to share her knowledge and kindness, her neighbors started to refer to her as the "Animal Advocate of the Neighborhood." Though she was humbled by the title, Viva was grateful for the opportunity to be of service to her community.

As the school bell rang for the final time, Viva and Cathy walked out of the building arm in arm, they planned to spend the summer break together, preparing for the transition to University, attending orientation events, and exploring Cathy's new school campus. They had supported each other.

The day had arrived for Viva to leave, everyone was present, including Darlington, her mom gave her some advice, while Mr,Mrs. Oliver made sure everything was ready, Cathy had just finished applying some makeup on Viva's face,Derek couldn't believe his eyes, he thought he was dreaming.

So Viva, you're leaving for real!. He looked at her sister with a completely sad expression. Saying goodbye is always hard, but knowing that we will see each other again makes it easier.safe Journey my sweet sister.

Viva saw the pains in her brothers eyes as she went closer to hug him. I will always be there for you Buddy!. Cathy joined them, followed by Darlington and everyone. It was a very sad moment for everyone.

The beep from Mr. Mike's car interrupted them.as they all turned around. Viva! Jason called, he had been quiet since because a lot was going on his mind. " I will miss you so much." He stretched out his hand to hold Viva, he looked straight at her. " you can always call me if you need my help on anything."

"Darlington, I will miss you too, but I will call you when I get there. She hugged him and later bid them goodbyes and departed from there.

Viva, are you ready for today? Mr. Mike asked.

"Mr. Mike,I'm so excited, but also a little nervous," she admitted with a nervous smile.

Mr. Mike smiled reassuringly, " it's completely normal to feel that way, Viva. Trust me, everyone feels a mix of excitement and nerves on their first day, just try making new friends. Are you ready?."

Viva, nodded with all eagerness. " yes I am! Thank you so much for offering to drive me, it's means a lot to me."

"It's nothing, you can turn on the music if you want something to ease your mind. He said staring at the car stereo."

" Am okay, thanks."

Chapter Eight

"Viva how are you preparing for your new school, hope you're aware that you'll meet different people of different backgrounds, race , tribe and culture, out there in New York City."

"Yes mom, Mr. Peterson said that Netford university has a lot of Educational departments just like other schools in Valley town, he mentioned how conducive the Environment is, and I just can't wait."

"Your principal told me to prepare your documents by tomorrow and he also assured you of your safety. My baby has grown so big, my dear, make sure you'll be a good girl ." Mrs. Smith said with a sad face.

"Mom, I still have three weeks left, and I am no longer a kid, I can take good care of myself, so don't worry, I will do just fine."

"Caressing Viva's palm, she stared at her. " I will miss you so, so, so much sweetie."

"I will miss you too, she gave her mom a tight hug."

Today's Viva's last day of being a student of Wilmington High School , as she and Cathy packed up their lockers, she turned to Cathy with a bittersweet smile. "Can you believe we're leaving this place and heading for University?." her voice was filled with a mix of excitement and uncertainty.

Cathy sighed, her eyes misting up a bit, " I know, Viva. It's hard to believe that we won't be seeing these familiar hallways every day. I am also looking forward to the new experience and adventures that await us in our different Universities.."

Viva nodded, understanding her friend's emotions. " you're right, Cathy. Change is a part of life and we need to embrace it. We've had a great time in high school, and I know we'll create even more amazing memories as we grow, it doesn't matter the university we attend, we will forever be best friends."

As the school bell rang for the final time, Viva and Cathy walked out of the building arm in arm, they planned to spend the summer break together, preparing for the transition to University, attending orientation events, and exploring Cathy's new school campus. They had supported each other.

The day had arrived for Viva to leave, everyone was present, including Darlington, her mom gave her some advice, while Mr,Mrs. Oliver made sure everything was ready, Cathy had just finished applying some makeup on Viva's face,Derek couldn't believe his eyes, he thought he was dreaming.

So Viva, you're leaving for real!. He looked at her sister with a completely sad expression. Saying goodbye is always hard, but knowing that we will see each other again makes it easier.safe Journey my sweet sister.

Viva saw the pains in her brothers eyes as she went closer to hug him. I will always be there for you Buddy!. Cathy joined them, followed by Darlington and everyone. It was a very sad moment for everyone.

The beep from Mr. Mike's car interrupted them.as they all turned around. Viva! Jason called, he had been quiet since because a lot was going on his mind. " I will miss you so much." He stretched out his hand to hold Viva, he looked straight at her. " you can always call me if you need my help on anything."

"Darlington, I will miss you too, but I will call you when I get there. She hugged him and later bid them goodbyes and departed from there.

"Viva, are you ready for today?." Mr. Mike asked.

"Mr. Mike, I'm so excited, but also a little nervous." she admitted with a nervous smile.

Mr. Mike smiled reassuringly, " it's completely normal to feel that way, Viva. Trust me, everyone feels a mix of excitement and nerves on their first day, just try making new friends. Are you ready?."

Viva, nodded with all eagerness. " Yes I am!, Thank you so much for offering to drive me, it means a lot to me."

"It's nothing, you can turn on the music if you want something to ease your mind." He said, staring at the car stereo."

" Am okay, thanks."

As they drove to the airport, Mr. Mike engaged in some conversations to ease her nervousness, they talked about her goals and aspirations, the subject she was looking up to, and he even talked about his own university memories.

"Mr. Mike: Viva, what do you have passion for?" He turned to look at Viva's face.

"Well I have passion for animals and I am hoping to be an expert in treating and taking good care of them." She said hastily.

Mr. Mike: oh wow!, that's grea but it sounds unusual for someone coming from our town, where they are few veterinarians. The people had no choice than to depend on their little knowledge about animal health, learned from their ancestors. That's is why about 39% of domestic animals die every week . and it has been that way since which results in the deaths of many animals each day. He looked at Viva trying to understand her expression. viva, why are you so quiet? He asked.

"I was just wondering why the people from Valley town hates cats so much."

Mr. Mike: "That's a very good thought. It's a long story but I would make it short and clear. Back in the days there lived a king called King Albert, .."

"I know king Albert, his pictures are on the history hall of Wilmington school."

Mr: Mike: yes, king Albert had two wives and two daughters, princess Sarah and Rachel but he never had a son, King Albert first wife, Queen Leah. Was barren for 21 years and 3 months, but Later gave birth to twin boys, Prince Samuel and Samson.

The second wife, Queen Stella. Was not happy for the news she heard. She became bittered and wanted to kill the newly born princes,she had a cat named Tom,which had trained to behave bad.

The king loved his children so much, but he loved the princes more. He gave most of his love and attention to the twins, one evening the king was having a feast and ordered that his first wife should prepare the meal instead of the palace maids. The king had always loved Queen Leah's delicious food. So this time he wanted to show not just his friends his friends, but the whole world how delicious his wife food tastes. So he invited the whole town and neighboring communities.

The time has arrived for the people to enjoy the delicious meal prepared by Queen Leah , the maid serves the specially made dish to the guests. After some minutes, the people scattered the food in the hall, the king was Aghast not knowing what the problem would have been.

Servant 1: " My Lord!!! …Tthere is cat dung in the meal My Queen prepared."

The king got so angry and told the servant to calm the people down, while they prepared another food.

Servant 2: " My Lord!. Tom. Queen Stella's Cat had made everywhere a mess."

The king ordered his servants to search everywhere for Tom. They couldn't find him, because Queen Stella had hidden him in an secret underground chamber. The king got so angry and Ordered his servants to annihilate all the cats in Valley town forever, he was so upset and ashamed of himself, the king of suhba, approached him, he was one of the most rich and powerful kings.

King Richard: "Albert!, did you just call me here to embarrass me?."

King Albert saw the Anger in his eyes and started Apologizing. " I am so, so, so, sorry! King Richard, that has never been my intentions, I was really hoping for everyone to rejoice with me, it things got really weird, this has never happened before, I just know what to do."

King Richard: I heard the cat's is from your palace, how would you have a cat in your palace that ruin everything, this is a very big embarrassment to you, take a look at the crowds leaving with anger, many of them traveled miles just for you and you ended everything with this?, better find a way to fix this, kill that cat, he doesn't deserve to live.

King Albert: I have ordered for it to be killed and If they don't find it then they should kill all the cats in the town and no cat would ever be allowed in my town, I will set a new law that all cats should be banned from this town or killed, henceforth; there shall be no cats in Valley town.

The next day rumors were everywhere that, the king gathered together just to give them a cat's dung to eat, to show how much he hated the people. When the king heard of it he gathered the people and Apologized to each of them he even send out Apology letters to those staying farther from the town, and then he made the official announcement that there shall not be found any cats in the town ever again! And it was sealed!.

The car wheels finally stopped. Mr. Mike stopped talking, but viva was curious to know if there's any way to remove the sealed law, that had been for many years.

" Mr. Mike. Do you think there's any way out?" She asked curiously.

"My dear I don't know, all I know right now is that we are at the airport, it's 6:00 am already and your flight will be leaving 6:30 am, so we don't have much time left, but I promise you, I will find out if there's a way to remove that old law."

Viva was a bit relaxed. "but Mr. Mike had a point there, I will do my own research too." She thought within herself, we needed to be prompt." As she glanced through the window she saw a lot of people in the airport, "it's just past six in the morning, and everywhere looks crowded." She wondered.

"Viva!. What are you doing?, come out!."

Viva said a brief prayers in her mind before she opened the door. She had never been to the airport before and she was excited at the same time, taking pictures of everything she saw at the airport.

An announcement was finally made for the next flight to takeoff .

Mr.Mike gave Viva some advice and encouragements before he left. Viva joined the others in the plane. She was very nervous, since it's her time on the plane, she sat quietly and as some announcements were made.

"Good morning Ladies and Gentlemen, Welcome onboard, this flight to New York City, my name is Luke Arvin and i am your In-flight service Director. Your Cabin crew are here to ensure you have an enjoyable flight to New York City this morning. Please put on your seat belt."

The announcement was clear, so Viva put on her seat belt, she now felt more relaxed than ever. As she made herself comfortable, she stare through the window to see how the plane had to move fast on land before it took off on air. She had never imagined she would be in a plane." Dad I promise to make you and mom proud of me." She said in a very low voice as she touched the necklace her father bought for her when he was still alive. Another announcement interrupted her, this time it's the Entertainment service.

" For enjoyment during our flight today, we have placed a complimentary copy of our In-flight magazine, pacific way, in the seat pocket in front of you. If you wish please feel free to take this with you when you leave.Those interested in buying duty free goods will also find our sky-shop brochure in the seat pocket. If you are in the first or business class sections, you will find controls for your reading flight, call button and the In-flight entertainment system on the inside of your armrest. In the economy cabin, these controls are located on your top seat armrest. To adjust your seat, push the round button beside the panel. Toilets for passengers seated in the economy cabins are located at the front, middle and rear of these cabins. Tea, coffee and a full bar service will be available Throughout the flight. If you require any special assistance, please contact the flight attendant nearest to you. We are here to ensure you have a comfortable and enjoyable flight. Later on we'll dim the cabin lights so you can get some rest. We recommend that while asleep, you keep your seatbelt fastened over the top of your blanket.

Chapter Nine

This way it will not be necessary to wake you up if the seatbelt sign comes on during the flight. If you don't want to wake up for breakfast, please advise the flight attendant. Thank you."

After hearing the announcements, Viva tightened her seatbelt and sat down quietly. She drank some coffee, Listened to music and finally fell asleep. After 2hrs,15 mins a farewell announcement woke Viva up, she sat up.

"We hope you have enjoyed the In-flight entertainment. We are now preparing to land. The bar is closed and we will soon collect your headset. May I remind you to complete your arrival and immigration documents by the time we arrive.
Ladies and gentlemen, now we are approaching New York City where the local time is 10: 04 am. At this stage you should be in your seat with your seat belt fastened. Personal television screens, footrests and seat tables must be stowed away and all hand luggage stored either in the overhead lockers or under the seat in front. Please ensure all electronic devices including laptop computer, computer games are turned off."

The plane finally stopped. Viva could feel the butterflies in her stomach grow stronger. "This was it- a new city, a new school, and a brand new chapter of my life." She made her way through the bustling airport, she scanned the crowds for someone holding a sign of her name on it, she quickly saw a tall man with a smile, holding a sign that said 'Welcome Viva Smith' she couldn't help but to feel a wave of relief wash over her.

"Are you Viva Smith?" He asked with a kind and friendly voice.

"Yes , that's me ." She replied,returning his smile.

As they made their way to the car, Mr. Jude immediately put her at ease with his charming conversation. He asked her about her interest, hometown and what I hope to achieve in Netford University. His Genuine interest in getting to know her made her feel comfortable and excited about her Journey ahead.

During the Drive to the school, Mr. Jude shared some interesting anecdotes about the city and its landmarks, painting a vivid picture of the vibrant community she was about to become a part of. Her excitement mounted, and she couldn't wait to start a new academic journey.

Upon reaching the school premises, Mr. Jude. gave her a tour of the campus, showcasing the classrooms, library, sports facilities and everything in between. He also introduced her to the staff members who would be there to support her throughout her time in Netford University.

As she stepped foot into the bustling hallways of Netford university, she couldn't help but feel a mix of nervousness and excitement. Being an international student was a new experience for her and she wasn't sure of what to expect. However, she knew deep down that she was ready for this new chapter of her life.

After the tour, Mr. Jude escorted her to her new hostel, where she would be living for the duration of her studies. He helped her settle into her room and show her where to find essential amenities like the study area, common room and cafeteria. His attention to detail and friendly demeanor made her feel right at home.

As days went by, she familiarized herself with the class. In each class, she met new classmates who welcomed her with warmth and kindness, they introduced her to other students, invited her to group study sessions and eagerly shared their experiences of being part of Netford University.

One of the first friends she made was Grace, a cheerful and outgoing girl from Nigeria, Who sat next to her in English class. They quickly discovered their shared love for animals.

In the Campus she made a group of friends, among which was Alex, a telented athlete from London, who was always up for a game of soccer during his free time. He had a contagious enthusiasm that brought smiles to everyone's faces. Sophie, on the other hand, was an artistic one in the group. She had a natural talent for painting from South Africa, and they spent countless afternoons capturing the beauty of the campus through her art work.

She met new students from different backgrounds and cultures and with each person her understanding of the world expanded. They bonded over shared experiences, laughed together and supported each other through ups and downs.

All the while, Mr. Jude remained a constant pillar of support. He often checked up on them, making sure they are settling well and offering guidance when needed. He wasn't just the person who picked her up from the airport, he became her friend and her mentor. always there to lend an ear or provide insightful advice.

Back home she had missed her family dearly including Cathy and Jason. She started calling them and chatting with them on social media asking Maxy her cat. She had missed her cat so much but she was sure he was in good care. she can't help but to tell them everything that had happened excluding nothing. She had always dreamt of pursuing a degree in veterinary medicine and she has not stopped nor slack back.

Darlington called her often to check up on her, he had recently been promoted in his company, he couldn't hold back the good news from Viva, he was so excited, and when Viva heard the good news, she was so happy for him.

Cathy also called telling her about how she had been enjoying the company of her new friend Jennifer.

One Tuesday morning, Mrs. Smith and Derek called her, telling her some very bad news.

Mrs. Smith: my dear are you done with your examinations?

" Not yet mom, the examinations had been postponed, we were given more time to prepare though one of our Lecturer's wives got diagnosed with cancer, she is a very good woman and everyone loved her. An announcement was made that she would be going for surgery. We even made donations for her, mom!. I pray the surgery goes smoothly."

Mrs. Smith: " I am sorry for your lecturer's wife, I believe she will get better if she gets the best treatment for her. Continue praying for her, we will do the same here. My dear Maxy is very sick, I gave him some drugs my friend told me about, but he is not getting better, I don't know what to do."

"Maxy is sick!!!.. oh mom, I know you must have been stressed out but you shouldn't have given him drugs without the doctor's recommendation." She said as she opened the curtains of her window.

Mrs. Smith: " You know it's really hard to find a veterinary clinic in Valley Town, I even went to Wilson town and the doctors were not available at the moment so I was so worried."

"It's okay mom, you should have called me earlier and I will direct you to some veterinary clinic outside Valley Town where I used to volunteer back then. But I will have to contact them."

Derek: Maxy's sickness was a sudden and worrisome turn of events for us, viva help us out please.

"It's okay Derek, Mom!, I will call Dr. Scott now and tell him about Maxy's condition."

Mrs: Smith: take good care of yourself, dear.

"You too mom, Derek please take care of mom."

Derek: Sure, I will, bye…

"Bye."

Viva Dial Dr. Scott's number and told him about Maxy's condition and Dr. Scott booked an appointment for Mrs. Smith and Derek to come to the clinic by noon.

Maxy was taken to the clinic, Dr. Scott and his team worked diligently to treat Maxy. Providing him with the best care possible, They gave him medication.

After the school examinations, she decided to go home and at least stay around and check up on Maxy. She can't wait to catch up with her Family, neighbors and friends. As he opened the door, she slowly walked in towards her mom's room.

Mrs: Smith: oh my goodness!, my baby girl you're home; you look so big now. She said as she hugged Viva so tight.

Oh mom I miss you every single day, how is everything?, where's Jason?. She turned around to see if Derek was inside the house.

Mrs. Smith: I am fine my dear and Derek is probably at the Mrs Sharon house, playing basketball with his friends. Derek has become a prominent young man.

"I know my buddy would have been a fully grown man now " she said , trying to imagine how big her brother would have been.

Mrs. Smith: Sweetheart I made some food for you , I know you will be very tired, so go watch up and come eat.

"I have really missed your delicious food, but how's Maxy's health?."

Mrs: Smith: Maxy is still at the clinic, Dr. Scott said Maxy has a critical sickness called FeLv, although he hasn't explained the meaning of FeLv.

FeLv! Oh my poor Maxy!, he must have been really suffering. FeLv is a ' feline Leukemia Virus, it's a viral infection that weakens the immune system, making cats susceptible to other diseases and infections. But don't worry mom, I will check on him Tomorrow.

Mr. Smith: Now I understand, let me call Darek to inform him that you're here.

No mom. don't bother him, let him enjoy himself. She said as she climbed the stairs.

Mrs. Smith: If you say so.

After eating she decided to pay Cathy a visit, as she walked through the familiar streets of her neighborhood, memories flooded back, reminding her of the countless adventures she and Cathy had shared. She felt like no time had passed at all.

When she reached her doorstep, she couldn't contain the excitement. She rang the doorbell and within a seconds, Cathy opened the door, greeting her with a big smile and hug. Cathy had missed Viva so much, they settled in her living room, surrounded by warm colors and photos documenting their years of friendship. They reminisce and laugh about their days at Wilmington school, recalling the pranks they pulled, the late night study sessions, and dreams they had shared. Catching up on everything that had transpired since they last saw each other. Viva shared tales of her university experience and wonderful animals she had encountered. She told Cathy about her veterinary class in New York and the incredible lectures she had met. They both marveled on how they had grown, yet they still feel like their teenage selves when they were together.

Before saying goodbyes, Cathy looked at Viva earnestly. "Viva, no matter where life takes us, I want you to remember that I will always be here for you." They hugged each other and Cathy promised to stop by at Viva's house to join them in Visiting Maxy at the Clinic tomorrow.

When Viva got home, she opened the door and stepped inside the house. She found Derek at the kitchen, looking slightly tired but with a smile on his face he greeted and hugged Viva so tight.

Derek: Welcome back, how was New York?

It was amazing Derek! So much to see and do. But what about you? How have things been here?.

Derek: Well it was quite an adventure taking care of Mom and Maxy. But don't worry, I managed everything just like you would have.

Viva's heart was filled with gratitude. " Derek you didn't have to do all these things on your own, you've been doing an incredible job taking care of mom, I am really proud of you, You're the best."

Derek: hey! Family is everything, Viva I knew you would have done the same for me if the roles were reversed. I just wanted to help out and make things easier for everyone while you were away.

Wiping tears of gratitude. " You truly are amazing Derek, I am so lucky to have you as my brother. Thank you so much for your endless support and devotion."

Derek smiled warmly. " It's what family does, Viva. We're in this together and I will be here for you, mom and Maxy, no matter what, now let's catch up on everything you missed in New York and tell me about all the exciting things you did!.

Chapter Ten

Mrs. Smith joined them as they delved into a beautiful evening of storytelling, laughter and cherished memories. Together they continue supporting one another.

Immediately it was afternoon. Viva, Derek and Cathy piled into the car and embarked on a short journey to the vet clinic, the clinic was some kilometers away from their town, the clinic walls were painted in soft pastel colors and vibrant artwork, providing a calming ambiance for both the furry animals and human patients. They saw some veterinarians on duty, the friendly receptionist greeted them warmly and assured them that Dr. Scott will attend to them soon.

After 5 minutes the receptionist told them to go inside Dr. Scott's office. Dr Scott welcomed them with a smile, and told them to have their seats.

Dr. Scott: Viva good to see you again. He smirked.

"Am happy to see you too, Dr. Scott." Viva replied.

Dr. Scott: So Viva can you introduce me to this Enthralling, Charming young lady because its seems she is the only one here that I don't know." He turned to Cathy, looking at her with a smile.

"My Apologies Dr.Scott, I would like you to meet my best friend Cathy and Cathy meet Dr. Scott."

He stood up to shake Cathy with a pleasant smile. " Nice to meet you Cathy."

"The pleasures are all mine Dr. Scott." she replied shyly.

Dr.Scott: you can address me as Scott, by the way I love to dress.

Cathy: oh thank you so much Scott, I got them from the Amazon store online. She replied blushing.

Dr. Scott: Oh I see, Amazon is one of the best places to buy anything, and their services are top notch. Don't worry everyone, my assistant is bringing Maxy.

Dr. Scott's Assistant brought Maxy inside the office,from the other entrance door of the office and placed him on the extra table beside the window. " meow" maxy interrupted them as the Assistant tried to make him lay on the table by holding his legs, maxy was so weak that he laid helplessly. Viva, Derek and Cathy rushed to meet him, Viva stretched out her hands carefully to carry maxy.

"Oh my baby has lost so much weight," she carried maxy on her body, she had missed him so much, she held him gently and placed him on her laps and comforted him with her touch and soothing words. Maxy's eyes met hers, his trust and gratitude shining through even in his weakened state. It was as if he understood that she was trying everything in her power to help him. As she stroked his fur and whispered sweet words, she could feel the depth of his bond with maxy.

The Veterinary team continued their efforts, using all their expertise to ease Maxy's suffering. They never gave up, showing immense compassion and dedication. With their help and Viva's unwavering love, Maxy's pain began to subside, allowing him to find moments of peace in his final hours.

In those precious moments together, Viva reminisced about all the joy Maxy had brought into her life. She remembered his playful antics, gentle purrs and comforting presence during her toughest days. She thanked Maxy for being her loyal companion, grateful for the beautiful memories they created together.

Dr. Scott: Viva we really tried our best, but we will still see if there's anything we can do, Dr. Scott assured.

"I know FeLv is a very bad sickness but I wish I was there for him when he needed me most. His condition couldn't have been this worse." She felt deep pain for her pets.

Derek: Viva; it's not your fault Maxy's condition got worse and you don't have to blame yourself for anything, it would have been better if there were good veterinary clinics in our town. I think all animals deserve good health and treatment, they deserve it Viva!.

Tears were rolling down Derek's eyes as he went closer to Viva, they hugged and comforted each other. " you're right Derek, all animals deserve a good and healthy life, they need to be cared for." Maxy's meow interrupted them again but this time in a very low voice, his body began to weaken, Maxy's spirit remained strong. As he peacefully drifted off to sleep, his breath slowed with each passing moment, Viva held him close. It was a bittersweet goodbye, but she found Solace in the knowledge that Maxy would no longer suffer.

Maxy's memories lived in their hearts, while his physical presence may have been absent, the love and warmth continued to surround her. She honored his memory by cherishing the time she was with him and by sharing his story with others, reminding them of the incredible bond that can exist between pets and humans.

Upon graduating from Netford University, Viva returned to her hometown and was eager to give back to the community that had shaped her. She opened her own Veterinary Clinic, combining her passion for animals with a commitment to provide compassionate and quality care to pets and their owners.

She continued to foster a strong bond with her family and friends, often visiting them during breaks and updating them on her progress. It's brought her immense joy to see Derek living his Dream as well. As years went by, she saw herself not just as a veterinarian but also a mentor to young aspiring Veterinarians, she dedicated her time visiting local schools, sharing her journey and inspiring others to pursue their passion in the field of veterinary medicine. In time, a new law was finally made that cats can now live in Valley town freely without being hurt or killed. Viva taught students the importance of having a pet and caring for them. The journey was filled with ups and downs but with the help of her family and friends made all the difference for her. She held a seminar in order to address the people of her town who love animals, and the turn up was massive.

Good day Ladies and gentlemen!. Thank you for giving me the opportunity to address you today as an animal lover, as someone who is deeply passionate about animals and their well-being, I'd like to share a few important things with all of you.
First and foremost, let's remember that animals deserve our respect, kindness and care. They are sentient beings with emotions, just like us. Every action we take, whether big or small, can make a significant impact on their lives. It is crucial for us to advocate for and support animal welfare organizations and initiatives. These organizations work tirelessly to rescue abused and abandoned animals, provide them with medical care and find them loving homes. By supporting them, whether through donations, volunteering or raising awareness, we contribute to their life-saving mission.
Education also plays a pivotal role in our efforts to protect and preserve animal welfare. teaching younger generations about the importance of empathy, responsible pet ownership and a compassionate world. Let's inspire curiosity and a love for animals within our children, nurturing the understanding of their vital role in the ecosystem.
Additionally, we must recognize the impact of our personal choices on the lives of animal welfare. Every decision we make has the potential to create a more compassionate and humane world for animals.
Lastly, Let's never underestimate the power of our voices. Advocating for stronger animal laws, speaking out against animal cruelty and promoting ethical treatment of animals can make substantial difference. By using social media platforms, and engaging in respectful discussions, we can mobilize change and protect the voiceless.
In conclusion as animal lovers, it's our duty to protect and care for those who cannot do so themselves. Together, let's make a commitment to prioritize animal welfare in our lives and

ensure that future generations inherit a world that cherishes and respects all creatures. Thank you.

The audience clapped, cheerfully. After the talk, Mr. Mike approached Viva with a warm smile on his face, he expressed how impressed he was for Viva's passion and knew about animal welfare and how he had shared a similar love for animals.

As a veterinarian, Viva days were filled with the joy of helping animals in need. It was during one of her busy days in the clinic that fate brought her face to face with the love of her life.

It was a hot summer afternoon when a distressed couple rushed into the clinic holding a small injured puppy in their arms. The puppy had been hit by a car, and they were desperate for immediate help. Without wasting a moment, Viva Sprang into action, gathering her team to provide emergency care for the little fur ball.

As they worked tirelessly to stabilize the puppy, Viva couldn't help but to notice a tall, kind-hearted man wearing a concerned expression standing at the back of the room. He introduced himself as Jason, and she immediately felt a connection, as if their souls had collided in that very moment. Throughout that day, Jason stayed by her side, his unwavering support and genuine concern for the puppy's well-being shining through.

Time seemed to fly by as they worked together to mend the puppy's broken bones and to tend to its injuries. Through it all, their conversations flowed effortlessly, filled with laughter, shared passion and a growing sense of familiarity.

Days turned into weeks, and the puppy now named Lucky, began to recover. Jason and Viva often found themselves bonding over the care and nurturing of Lucky. They took turns staying up throughout the night to monitor his progress, and during those quiet moments, their connection deepened.

As the days turned into months, Lucky's transformation was nothing short of miraculous. He went from a frail little pup to a bundle of energy, bouncing around the clinic transcended into deep and profound love that filled their souls. They continued to support each other in their respective careers, finding solace in each other's understanding and unwavering support. Jason's genuine love for animals perfectly complemented her passion for veterinary care and they often found themselves discussing cases and sharing their experiences, constantly learning from each other.

As time went on, they began to envision a future together. They dream of opening their own sanctuary, a place where they can provide loving homes for animals in need and educate the community about animal welfare. This shared vision brought them even closer, as they worked side by side to turn our dream into a reality. Together they poured their hearts and souls into building the sanctuary, dedicating their time, resources and love to creating a safe haven for animals. Their days were filled with laughter, hardwork and the fulfillment of knowing they were making a difference in the lives of those who couldn't speak for themselves.

The sanctuary soon became a thriving community hub, attracting volunteers, sponsors and supporters who shared their passion. Their love for animals and dedication to their well-being served as an inspiration to those around them. Amidst the chaos and responsibilities of running the sanctuary, their love continued to grow deeper. Jason's unwavering support and kindness touched her heart every single day. He is her rock, her best friend and the love of her life.

One beautiful evening, as the sun set over the sanctuary, Jason surprised viva with a romantic dinner. The air was filled with a sense of magic as he got down on his knee, opening a small velvet box to reveal the most stunning engagement ring she had ever seen. Tears of Joy streamed down her face as she wholeheartedly said "Yes!" . They sealed their love with a heartfelt kiss, knowing that their Journey together was just about to begin.

One warm summer day, surrounded by their loved ones . They exchanged vows of love and commitment. It was a day filled with joy, laughter, and celebration as they embarked on a new chapter as husband and wife.

Cathy also got married to her long time boyfriend David. While Derek got fully involved with his work, Viva and Jason, gave birth to a boy and a girl named Chris and Christine.
They lived happily ever after.

__THE END__

Things you should know

Cats

1. Common Illnesses: Cats can be prone to certain common illnesses, including urinary tract infections, dental disease, upper respiratory infections (URIs), gastrointestinal issues, and obesity.

2. Preventive Healthcare: Regular veterinary check-ups are crucial to catch and prevent any potential health issues early on. Vaccinations, flea and tick prevention, regular dental care, and deworming are all essential components of preventive healthcare for cats.

3. Signs of Illness: Cats are known for their ability to hide signs of illness, so it's important to be vigilant and watch for any changes in behavior. Common signs of sickness in cats include decreased appetite, changes in litter box habits, lethargy, hiding or isolation, vomiting, diarrhea, coughing, sneezing, or abnormal weight loss or gain.

4. Feline Lower Urinary Tract Disease (FLUTD): FLUTD is a common condition affecting the urinary system in cats. It can include disorders such as urinary tract infections, bladder stones, or even urinary blockages. Symptoms may include straining to urinate, frequent urination, blood in the urine, or urinating outside the litter box.

5. Dental Disease: Dental issues are prevalent in cats. Periodontal disease, gingivitis, and tooth decay can cause discomfort, bad breath, and can even lead to more serious health problems if left untreated. Regular dental cleanings and proper oral hygiene are important for a cat's overall health.

6. Feline Leukemia Virus (FeLV) and Feline Immunodeficiency Virus (FIV): These are two contagious viral diseases that can be transmitted between cats through close contact, such as fighting, mating, or sharing food and water bowls. Testing for and vaccinating against these viruses is essential, especially for cats that spend time outdoors or are at risk of exposure.

7. Parasites: Cats can be susceptible to parasites, including fleas, ticks, ear mites, and internal parasites like roundworms and tapeworms. Regular parasite prevention and deworming are important to keep your cat healthy.

8. Nutritional Needs: A well-balanced, species-appropriate diet is crucial for a cat's overall health. Feeding your cat high-quality cat food that meets their nutritional requirements helps support their immune system and can prevent certain health issues, such as obesity and digestive disorders.

9. Stress and Illness: Cats are sensitive creatures and can be prone to stress-related illnesses. Environmental changes, such as moving to a new home or the introduction of a new pet, can cause stress and lead to behavioral changes or physical ailments. Providing a calm and enriched environment can help minimize stress in your feline friend.

10. Senior Cat Care: As cats age, they become more susceptible to certain age-related health conditions like arthritis, kidney disease, and hyperthyroidism. Regular geriatric check-ups and providing appropriate care can help manage these conditions and ensure your senior cat remains happy and comfortable in their golden years.

11. Zoonotic Diseases: Some illnesses that affect cats can also be transmitted to humans, known as zoonotic diseases. Examples include toxoplasmosis, ringworm, and certain types of bacterial infections. Proper hygiene, handling, and regular handwashing after interacting with cats can help reduce the risk of transmission.

12. Vaccinations: Vaccinations are an essential part of preventive healthcare for cats. Core vaccines, such as those for feline panleukopenia (FPV), feline herpesvirus (FHV), and feline calicivirus (FCV), are recommended for all cats. Non-core vaccines, such as those for feline leukemia virus (FeLV) and rabies, may be given based on a cat's lifestyle and risk factors.

13. Dental Care: Just like humans, cats can develop dental problems, such as tartar buildup and gum disease. Regular teeth brushing, using a cat-specific toothpaste and toothbrush, helps maintain good oral hygiene and prevents dental issues. Additionally, providing dental treats or toys that promote chewing can also help keep your cat's teeth clean.

14. Litter Box Hygiene: Cleanliness is essential when it comes to your cat's litter box. Scoop the litter box daily to remove any waste and clumps. Also, remember to completely change the litter and thoroughly clean the box on a regular basis to prevent bacterial build-up and maintain your cat's litter box hygiene.

15. Safe Environment: Ensure your cat's environment is safe and free from hazards. Secure any toxic substances, such as cleaning products or certain plants, out of your cat's reach. Keep electrical cords tucked away or protected to prevent chewing. Also, provide vertical spaces like cat trees, shelves, or window perches for your cat to explore and feel secure.

16. Mental and Physical Enrichment: Cats need mental and physical stimulation to thrive. Provide interactive toys, puzzle feeders, and scratching posts to keep them mentally alert. Play with your cat regularly using toys to engage their natural hunting instincts and keep them physically active.

17. Grooming: Regular grooming helps maintain your cat's coat and overall hygiene. Brushing your cat helps remove loose fur, prevents matting, and reduces hairballs. Additionally, it allows you to check for any skin issues, fleas, or ticks.

18. Spaying/Neutering: Getting your cat spayed or neutered not only helps control the population but also offers numerous health benefits. Spaying female cats reduces the risk of uterine infections and mammary tumors, while neutering male cats helps prevent testicular cancer and reduces the likelihood of certain behavioral issues.

Dogs

1. Common Illnesses: Dogs can experience a range of common illnesses, including gastrointestinal issues like diarrhea and vomiting, skin infections or allergies, ear infections, urinary tract infections, dental problems, joint issues like arthritis, and infectious diseases such as parvovirus and kennel cough.

2. Signs of Illness: Dogs may show signs of illness such as decreased appetite, weight loss or gain, lethargy, coughing, sneezing, excessive panting, vomiting, diarrhea, changes in drinking or urination habits, limping, itching or redness in the skin, and changes in behavior. It's important to pay attention to these signs and consult a veterinarian if you notice anything concerning.

3. Preventative Care: Regular veterinary check-ups, vaccinations, and preventive measures are crucial to keeping your dog healthy. Vaccinations protect against common diseases like parvovirus, distemper, rabies, and kennel cough. Additionally, routine flea and tick prevention, heartworm prevention, and regular grooming can help maintain your dog's well-being.

4. Dental Health: Dental issues are prevalent in dogs, so maintaining good dental hygiene is important. Regular teeth brushing, providing dental chews or toys, and regular dental check-ups with your veterinarian can help prevent periodontal disease, tooth decay, and bad breath.

5. Parasite Control: Dogs are often susceptible to parasitic infestations, including fleas, ticks, and internal parasites like roundworms and hookworms. Regular preventive treatments are necessary to protect your dog from these parasites, as they can cause various health problems.

6. Exercise and Mental Stimulation: Regular exercise and mental stimulation are vital for a dog's overall health and well-being. Adequate physical activity helps maintain a healthy weight, strengthens their muscles and joints, and supports their mental health by reducing anxiety and boredom.

7. Good Nutrition: Providing a balanced and healthy diet is essential for your dog's health. Consult with your veterinarian to ensure you're feeding them a nutritionally appropriate diet based on their breed, age, and any specific health concerns they may have.

8. Allergies: Dogs can develop allergies to certain foods, environmental factors (such as pollen or dust mites), or fleas. Common allergy symptoms include itching, sneezing, watery eyes, and

skin irritation. Treatment may include identifying and avoiding the allergen, oral medications to alleviate symptoms, or immunotherapy to desensitize the dog's immune system to the allergen.

9. Bladder Infections: Bladder infections, caused by bacteria entering the urinary tract, can lead to frequent urination, pain or discomfort while urinating, and blood in the urine. Treatment usually involves a course of antibiotics prescribed by a veterinarian. Ensuring your dog has access to fresh water and regular bathroom breaks can also help prevent bladder infections.

10. Arthritis: Arthritis is a common condition in older dogs, causing joint inflammation and stiffness. Treatment options include pain management medications, joint supplements (such as glucosamine and chondroitin), weight management, physical therapy, and providing comfortable bedding and support. Additionally, gentle exercise can help improve mobility and strengthen muscles.

11. Digestive Issues: Digestive problems like diarrhea and vomiting can have various causes, such as dietary indiscretion, food allergies, or gastrointestinal infections. Treatment may involve dietary changes, probiotics, medications to relieve symptoms, and in severe cases, fluid therapy or hospitalization.

12. Respiratory Infections: Respiratory infections such as kennel cough and pneumonia can cause coughing, sneezing, difficulty breathing, and nasal discharge. Treatment may include rest, antibiotics, cough suppressants, and additional supportive care as directed by the veterinarian.

13. Dental Disease: Dental problems, such as gum disease and tooth decay, can be painful for dogs and can lead to complications if left untreated. Regular dental care, including daily teeth brushing and annual professional cleanings, can help prevent dental disease. Treatment may include dental scaling, extractions, and antibiotics if there is an infection.

14. Eye Infections: Dogs can develop eye infections from various causes, such as bacteria, viruses, or foreign objects. Symptoms may include redness, discharge, squinting, or cloudiness. Treatment may involve regular cleaning, antibiotic eye drops, or ointments, depending on the severity and underlying cause. It's important to consult with a veterinarian for proper diagnosis and treatment.

15. Skin Infections: Skin infections in dogs can result from allergies, mites, fungal infections, or underlying conditions. Symptoms may include itching, redness, hair loss, or sores. Treatment options may include medicated shampoos, topical ointments, oral medication, and addressing any underlying issues, such as allergies or parasites.

16. Ear Infections: Dogs, particularly those with long and floppy ears, are prone to ear infections. Common signs include head shaking, scratching at the ears, odor, discharge, or redness. Treatment may involve ear cleaning, medication (such as ear drops), and managing

any underlying factors contributing to the infection. Regular ear cleaning can help prevent future infections.

17. Heartworm Disease: Heartworm disease is a serious and potentially fatal condition caused by parasitic worms. Prevention is crucial, and there are various options available, including monthly oral or topical medications prescribed by a veterinarian. Treatment for heartworm disease can be complex and might include medications, exercise restrictions, and, in severe cases, hospitalization.

18. Kennel Cough: Kennel cough, also known as infectious tracheobronchitis, is a highly contagious respiratory infection often seen in dogs that have been in close proximity to other dogs, such as in boarding facilities or dog parks. Symptoms include a persistent cough, sneezing, nasal discharge, and sometimes fever. Treatment may involve rest, cough suppressants, antibiotics, and sometimes supportive care like fluids or nebulization.

19. Urinary Tract Infections (UTIs): UTIs can occur in dogs, causing frequent urination, blood in urine, discomfort, or accidents in the house. Bacterial UTIs can be treated with a course of antibiotics prescribed by a veterinarian. Ensuring your dog has access to plenty of fresh water, regular potty breaks, and a balanced diet can help prevent UTIs.

20. Arthritis: Arthritis is a degenerative joint disease commonly seen in senior dogs but can also affect younger dogs due to genetic predisposition or injury. Symptoms include stiffness, lameness, difficulty getting up, and reluctance to play or exercise. Treatment options may include pain medication, joint supplements, weight management, physical therapy, and alternative therapies like acupuncture or laser therapy.

21. Diabetes: Diabetes mellitus is a metabolic disorder resulting from the body's inability to regulate blood sugar levels. Signs include increased thirst, frequent urination, weight loss, and lethargy. Treatment involves insulin therapy, diet management, and regular monitoring of blood sugar levels. It's crucial to work closely with a veterinarian to ensure proper insulin dosage and management.

22. Allergies: Dogs can develop allergies to various environmental factors, such as pollen, dust mites, or certain foods. Common signs of allergies include itching, redness, skin irritation, ear infections, or gastrointestinal upset. Treatment may involve allergen avoidance, a hypoallergenic diet, allergy testing, and medications like antihistamines or steroids to manage symptoms.

Rabbits

1. Gastrointestinal Stasis: This condition occurs when a rabbit's digestive system slows down or stops entirely. Symptoms include reduced or no appetite, decreased fecal output, lethargy, and abdominal bloating. Treatment may involve fluid therapy, pain management, syringe feeding, and encouraging movement to stimulate digestion. It's important to address the underlying causes, such as dental issues, dietary imbalances, or stress.

2. Dental Problems: Rabbits have continuously growing teeth, and if they are not properly worn down through chewing on hay and other fibrous materials, dental issues such as overgrowth, spurs, or abscesses can occur. Signs of dental problems include drooling, decreased appetite, weight loss, and reluctance to eat hard foods. Treatment often involves dental filing or trimming under anesthesia, pain management, and addressing any concurrent infections.

3. Respiratory Infections: Rabbits can develop respiratory infections caused by bacteria, viruses, or parasites. Symptoms may include sneezing, nasal discharge, labored breathing, and lethargy. Treatment typically includes antibiotics, supportive care, and environmental changes to minimize dust and other irritants.

4. Ear Mites: These tiny parasites can cause itching, head shaking, ear discharge, and even ear canal inflammation in rabbits. Treatment involves veterinary examination and ear cleaning, as well as prescribed medications to eliminate the mites.

5. Flystrike: This is a serious condition where flies lay eggs on a rabbit's soiled fur, and the resulting maggots can cause deep tissue damage and infection. Prevention involves diligent hygiene and close monitoring, especially in warmer months. Treatment includes prompt removal of maggots, wound care, and antibiotics to control infection.

6. Heat Stress: Rabbits are sensitive to high temperatures and can suffer from heat stroke. Signs include excessive panting, lethargy, and collapse. Immediate cooling measures, such as moving the rabbit to a cool, shaded area and using damp towels, are crucial, along with veterinary assessment.

7. Regularly grooming your rabbit, especially those with long fur, can help prevent issues such as hairballs and matting. It's also an excellent opportunity to check for any skin abnormalities, injuries or signs of parasites.

8. Providing your rabbit with a stimulating and enriching environment is crucial for their mental and physical well-being. Offer a variety of safe toys, tunnels, and platforms for them to explore, as well as opportunities for supervised playtime outside of their enclosure.

9. Gentle and regular handling can help your rabbit become more accustomed to human interaction, reducing stress and fear. However, it's essential to approach handling with patience and respect for your rabbit's comfort level.

10. Maintaining a clean living environment for your rabbit is vital in preventing health issues such as flystrike and respiratory problems. Regularly clean and disinfect their living space, provide fresh bedding, and ensure access to clean water and a balanced diet.

Chickens

1. Coccidiosis: This is a common parasitic disease that affects the intestinal tract of chickens, often caused by unsanitary living conditions. Symptoms include diarrhea, decreased appetite, lethargy, and in severe cases, blood in the stool. Prevention and treatment involve maintaining a clean coop, providing medicated feed, and using anticoccidial medications as directed by a veterinarian.

2. Marek's Disease: This is a viral disease that can cause tumors, paralysis, and eventually death in chickens. Symptoms include paralysis, weight loss, and a change in behavior. Preventative measures include vaccination, and unfortunately, there's no cure once a chicken is infected.

3. Respiratory infections: Chickens can suffer from respiratory illnesses caused by bacteria, viruses, or environmental factors. Symptoms include coughing, sneezing, nasal discharge, and difficulty breathing. Treatment may involve antibiotics, proper ventilation in the coop, and limiting exposure to drafts and dust.

4. Egg binding: This occurs when a hen is unable to pass an egg, which can be a life-threatening condition. Symptoms include lethargy, fluffed feathers, and straining. Treatment may involve gently massaging the abdomen to help the hen expel the egg, along with providing supplemental calcium.

5. Bumblefoot: This is a common bacterial infection in a chicken's foot caused by injury or unsanitary conditions. Symptoms include swelling, redness, and lameness. Treatment involves cleaning the affected foot, removing any scabs, and applying antibiotics and bandaging as needed.

6. Quarantine new birds: If you introduce new birds to your flock, it's crucial to quarantine them for a few weeks to prevent the spread of diseases. This allows you to monitor their health and ensure they are free from any contagious illnesses before integrating them with the rest of the flock.

7. Provide a balanced diet: A well-balanced diet is essential for maintaining your chickens' overall health and resistance to illness. Ensure they have access to quality feed appropriate for their age and nutritional needs. Additionally, offering occasional treats such as fresh fruits and vegetables can help support their immune system.

8. Monitor flock behavior: Regularly observe your flock for any changes in behavior, eating habits, or appearance. Early detection of illness can significantly improve the chances of successful treatment.

9. Practice good biosecurity: Implementing good biosecurity measures, such as controlling access to your coop, disinfecting equipment, and limiting contact with other flocks, can help prevent the introduction and spread of diseases.

10. Consult a poultry veterinarian: If you notice any concerning symptoms or have questions about your chickens' health, it's best to seek advice from a veterinarian experienced in poultry care. They can provide personalized recommendations and treatment options based on your flock's specific needs.

Hamster

1. Wet tail (proliferative ileitis): Symptoms include wet and soiled fur around the tail area, lethargy, and diarrhea. Treatment may involve antibiotics, fluid therapy, and supportive care.

2. Respiratory infections: Symptoms include sneezing, coughing, nasal discharge, and labored breathing. Treatment may involve antibiotics, maintaining a warm and clean environment, and providing proper ventilation.

3. Mites and external parasites: Symptoms include excessive scratching, hair loss, and skin irritation. Treatment may involve medication to eliminate the parasites and thoroughly cleaning the hamster's living environment.

4. Diabetes: Symptoms include excessive thirst, weight loss, and increased urination. Treatment may involve dietary changes, medication (as prescribed by a veterinarian), and monitoring blood sugar levels.

5. Tumors: Symptoms may include visible lumps or masses on the body. Treatment may involve surgical removal of the tumor, if possible, and supportive care.

6. Dental problems: Symptoms include drooling, difficulty eating, and overgrown teeth. Treatment may involve filing or trimming overgrown teeth, providing appropriate chew toys, and adjusting the diet to aid in dental wear.

7. Diarrhea: Symptoms include loose or watery stools. Treatment may involve identifying and addressing the underlying cause, providing a bland diet, and ensuring adequate hydration.

8. Constipation: Symptoms include difficulty passing stools. Treatment may involve adjusting the diet to include more fiber, providing access to fresh water, and, if necessary, gentle massages to aid in relieving the constipation.

9. Abscesses: Symptoms include swelling, redness, and pain at the site of the abscess. Treatment may involve draining the abscess, providing antibiotics, and keeping the affected area clean.

10. Dehydration: Symptoms include sunken eyes, lethargy, and dry or tacky mucous membranes. Treatment involves providing access to fresh water and, if necessary, offering rehydration solutions as directed by a veterinarian.

11. Overgrown nails: Symptoms include excessively long or curled nails. Treatment involves regular nail trimming to prevent discomfort and potential injury to the hamster.

12. Heatstroke: Symptoms include rapid breathing, weakness, and disorientation. Treatment involves moving the hamster to a cooler environment, providing access to water, and, if necessary, gently cooling the hamster with a damp cloth.

13. Stroke: Symptoms may include sudden paralysis, loss of balance, or disorientation. Unfortunately, there is no specific treatment for a stroke in hamsters, so providing a quiet and comfortable environment, as well as supportive care, is essential.

14. Eye infections: Symptoms include redness, discharge, and squinting. Treatment may involve cleaning the affected eye, using saline solution, and administering antibiotic eye drops, if prescribed by a veterinarian.

15. Traumatic injuries: Symptoms may vary depending on the nature of the injury, but treatment generally involves addressing the specific injury, providing pain relief, and protecting the hamster from further harm.

Parrots

1. Respiratory infections: Symptoms may include sneezing, coughing, nasal discharge, and labored breathing. Treatment can involve antibiotics, maintaining a warm and clean environment, and providing proper ventilation.

2. Psittacosis (parrot fever): Symptoms can include respiratory issues, lethargy, and diarrhea. Treatment generally involves antibiotics, isolation from other birds, and thorough cleaning of the living environment.

3. Nutritional deficiencies: Symptoms may include feather abnormalities, poor growth, and general weakness. Treatment involves correcting the diet, potentially supplementing with vitamins and minerals, and ensuring access to a varied and balanced diet.

4. Feather plucking: This behavior can be a sign of stress, boredom, or underlying health issues. Treatment may involve addressing potential causes, providing enrichment, and, in some cases, working with a veterinarian to rule out medical reasons for the behavior.

5. Bumblefoot: This condition involves swelling and sores on the feet caused by pressure or infection. Treatment may involve antibiotics, cleaning the affected area, and improving perching surfaces and environmental conditions.

6. Gastrointestinal issues: Symptoms may include diarrhea, undigested food in the feces, and decreased appetite. Treatment may involve dietary adjustments, probiotics, and addressing potential causes such as parasites or bacterial overgrowth.

7. Beak and feather disease: This viral disease can cause feather abnormalities and beak deformities. Unfortunately, there is no cure, so treatment focuses on supportive care and preventing the spread of the virus to other birds.

8. Egg binding: This occurs when a female bird is unable to pass an egg. Treatment may involve providing a warm and humid environment, gentle massage, and, in severe cases, veterinary assistance to manually remove the egg.

9. Parasites: External parasites such as mites and lice can cause itching and discomfort. Treatment involves using appropriate avian-safe products to eliminate the parasites and thoroughly cleaning the bird's living environment.

10. Liver disease: Symptoms may include yellowing of the skin, weight loss, and lethargy. Treatment may involve dietary adjustments, medications, and addressing potential underlying causes such as poor diet or exposure to toxins.

11. Aspergillosis: This fungal infection can cause respiratory distress and general illness. Treatment typically involves antifungal medications, improving environmental conditions to reduce the risk of fungal growth, and providing supportive care.

12. Preening issues: Overpreening or plucking feathers can lead to bald spots and skin irritation. Treatment involves addressing underlying causes, providing environmental enrichment, and possibly working with a veterinarian to manage any medical issues contributing to the behavior.

13. Wing injuries: This can include broken bones, sprains, or cuts. Treatment may involve splinting, wound care, and providing a safe and quiet environment for healing.

14. Pesticide exposure: Accidental exposure to toxic substances can cause a range of symptoms, including weakness, tremors, and seizures. Immediate treatment involves removing the bird from the source of contamination, thorough cleaning, and seeking emergency veterinary care.

15. Behavioral issues: Parrots can develop various behavioral problems due to stress, boredom, or improper socialization. Treatment involves addressing the underlying causes, providing mental stimulation, and potentially seeking the help of an avian behavior specialist.

Horse

1. Colic: Symptoms may include pawing, rolling, and signs of abdominal discomfort. Treatment involves immediate veterinary attention, potential pain management, and, in some cases, surgical intervention.

2. Laminitis: This condition causes inflammation in the hoof and can result in severe lameness. Treatment may involve anti-inflammatory medications, dietary adjustments, and farrier care to support the affected hooves.

3. Equine influenza: Symptoms can mimic human flu, including coughing, nasal discharge, and fever. Treatment may involve supportive care, including rest and isolation, and potentially vaccination to prevent future occurrences.

4. Equine herpesvirus (EHV): This virus can cause respiratory illness, abortion in pregnant mares, and neurological symptoms. Treatment involves supportive care, isolation of affected animals, and potentially vaccination to reduce the risk of infection.

5. Strangles: This highly contagious bacterial infection can cause fever, nasal discharge, and abscesses in the lymph nodes. Treatment may involve antibiotics, isolation of infected horses, and proper hygiene to prevent the spread of the disease.

6. Cushing's disease (PPID): Symptoms may include excessive drinking, weight loss, and changes in coat quality. Treatment involves medication to manage hormone imbalances, dietary adjustments, and regular veterinary monitoring.

7. Equine gastric ulcers: Symptoms may include poor appetite, weight loss, and signs of discomfort. Treatment involves medication to reduce stomach acid, dietary changes, and environmental modifications to reduce stress.

8. Skin conditions: Horses can develop a range of skin issues, such as rain rot, sweet itch, and dermatitis. Treatment may involve topical medications, fly control, and addressing potential underlying causes such as allergies or parasites.

9. Thrush: This bacterial infection affects the hooves, leading to a foul odor and black discharge. Treatment involves cleaning the affected area, applying antiseptic agents, and maintaining proper hoof hygiene.

10. Hoof abscesses: Symptoms can include sudden lameness and sensitivity to hoof testing. Treatment involves drainage of the abscess, poulticing the affected hoof, and providing pain relief as needed.

11. EPM (equine protozoal myeloencephalitis): This neurological disease can cause weakness, incoordination, and muscle atrophy. Treatment may involve antiprotozoal medications and supportive care to manage neurological symptoms.

12. Profuse bleeding: In cases of severe injury leading to profuse bleeding, immediate first aid is crucial. This may involve applying pressure to the wound, bandaging the affected area, and seeking prompt veterinary care for further treatment.

13. Rhabdomyolysis (tying-up): This condition involves muscle stiffness, reluctance to move, and dark urine. Treatment may include rest, electrolyte management, and addressing potential triggers such as exercise-related stress.

14. Choke: Symptoms include difficulty swallowing, drooling, and coughing. Treatment may involve veterinary intervention to clear the obstruction and provide supportive care to the affected horse.

15. Equine metabolic syndrome (EMS): This metabolic disorder can lead to obesity, insulin resistance, and laminitis. Treatment may involve dietary management, weight control, and monitoring for laminitis risk factors.

Fish

1. Ich (Ichthyophthirius multifiliis): This is a common parasitic infection causing white spots on fish. Treatment may involve raising the temperature, adding aquarium salt, and using medications specifically formulated to treat Ich.

2. Fin rot: This bacterial infection can cause fraying or disintegration of the fins. Treatment may involve improving water quality, addressing potential stressors, and using antibiotics if necessary.

3. Swim bladder disorder: This condition can lead to buoyancy issues and difficulty swimming. Treatment may involve feeding a diet with high fiber content, adjusting water parameters, and providing a stress-free environment for the affected fish.

4. Dropsy: This condition leads to swelling and fluid retention in the fish's body, causing bloating. Treatment may involve isolation, antibiotic medications, and maintaining optimal water quality to reduce stress on the affected fish.

5. Velvet disease (Oodinium): This is a parasitic infection causing a gold or rust-colored dusting on the fish's skin. Treatment may involve medications to eliminate the parasites and adjusting water parameters to reduce stress.

6. Popeye: This condition causes protruding eyes in fish due to infection or injury. Treatment may involve isolating the affected fish, addressing water quality issues, and using antibiotics under veterinary guidance.

7. Columnaris (Flexibacter columnaris): This bacterial infection can cause white patches on the fish's skin, mouth, or gills. Treatment may involve antibiotic medications, improving water quality, and isolating infected fish to prevent the spread of the disease.

8. Anchor worm: This parasite attaches to the fish's body, causing irritation and potential infection. Treatment may involve physically removing the anchor worm, medicating the affected fish, and addressing water quality to prevent further infestation.

9. Gill flukes: These external parasites can affect the fish's gills, leading to respiratory distress. Treatment may involve using medications specifically targeting gill flukes and improving water quality to reduce stress on the fish.

10. Fungal infections: Fish can develop fungal infections, typically appearing as white or gray cottony growths on the skin or fins. Treatment may involve antifungal medications, maintaining optimal water quality, and addressing potential stressors in the aquarium.

11. Dropsy: This condition causes abdominal swelling and fluid retention in fish. Treatment involves isolating the affected fish, improving water quality, and using antibacterial medications

12. Fish tuberculosis (Mycobacterium marinum): This bacterial infection can affect the internal organs of fish, leading to symptoms such as emaciation and internal lesions. Unfortunately, there is no effective treatment for fish tuberculosis, and affected fish may need to be euthanized to prevent the spread of the disease.

13. Hole in the head disease: This condition, also known as head and lateral line erosion (HLLE), can cause pitting and erosion on the fish's head and lateral line. Treatment may involve improving water quality, providing a balanced diet, and using medication to address potential bacterial or parasitic factors contributing to the condition.

14. Velvet disease (Amyloodinium): Similar to Oodinium, this parasitic infection causes a gold or rust-colored dusting on the fish's skin. Treatment may involve medications to eliminate the parasites and adjusting water parameters to reduce stress.

15. Dropsy: This condition leads to severe bloating and fluid retention in the fish, often resulting from underlying organ dysfunction. Treatment may involve isolating the affected fish, providing supportive care, and consulting with a veterinarian for potential treatment options.

Sheep

1. Footrot: This bacterial infection causes inflammation and lameness in the feet. Treatment may involve trimming overgrown hoof tissue and applying topical antibiotics, as well as improving hygiene to prevent further infections.

2. Internal parasites (e.g., worms): Sheep are susceptible to various internal parasites, which can cause weight loss, poor growth, and anemia. Treatment involves deworming with specific anthelmintic medications and implementing pasture management practices to reduce parasite load.

3. External parasites (e.g., lice and mites): Infestations of external parasites can lead to skin irritation and wool loss. Treatment includes applying insecticidal treatments, such as dips or sprays, and providing clean bedding to prevent re-infestation.

4. Scours (diarrhea): This condition can result from various causes, including infectious agents and dietary issues. Treatment involves maintaining adequate hydration, addressing nutritional imbalances, and administering appropriate medications if necessary.

5. Pneumonia: Respiratory infections can occur due to bacterial, viral, or environmental factors. Treatment includes providing warmth, isolation for affected animals, and administering antibiotics under veterinary guidance.

6. Mastitis: Inflammation of the udder can lead to reduced milk production and discomfort. Treatment involves antibiotic therapy, supportive care, and ensuring proper milking hygiene to prevent recurrence.

7. Enterotoxemia (overeating disease): This condition can occur when sheep consume excessive amounts of grain or lush pasture, leading to deadly toxins produced by Clostridium perfringens. Vaccination against enterotoxemia and managing diet changes are critical for prevention.

8. Pregnancy toxemia (ketosis): This metabolic disorder commonly affects pregnant ewes and can result from inadequate nutrition or stress. Treatment involves providing energy-dense feeds, supportive care, and potential induction of labor if necessary.

9. Bloat: An accumulation of gas in the rumen can cause bloating and discomfort. Treatment includes relieving gas buildup and addressing dietary factors that contribute to bloat, such as sudden changes in diet or access to lush forage.

10. Contagious ecthyma (scabby mouth): This viral infection causes lesions around the mouth and can affect young lambs. Treatment involves supportive care, managing secondary bacterial infections, and isolation to prevent the spread of the virus.

11. Foot abscess: Infections in the hoof can lead to abscess formation and discomfort. Treatment consists of draining the abscess, cleansing the affected area, and providing appropriate antibiotic therapy if necessary.

12. Polioencephalomalacia (PEM): This neurological disorder can result from thiamine deficiency or other causes. Treatment involves administering thiamine supplements and addressing underlying nutritional imbalances.

13. Ovine pulmonary adenocarcinoma (Jaagsiekte): This contagious viral tumor disease affects the lungs of sheep and can lead to respiratory distress. There is no specific treatment, and affected animals may need to be isolated to prevent spread within the flock.

14. Tetanus: This bacterial disease leads to muscle stiffness and spasms. Treatment includes administering tetanus antitoxin, wound care to prevent further contamination, and ensuring proper vaccination to prevent future cases.

15. External injuries: Sheep can suffer from various types of external injuries, such as cuts, abrasions, or fractures. Treatment involves cleaning and dressing wounds, providing pain relief, and potentially immobilizing fractures for proper healing.

Turtle

1. Respiratory Infections: Common signs include wheezing, discharge from the nose or mouth, and labored breathing. Treatment involves keeping the turtle's environment clean, providing proper basking and UVB lighting, and, in severe cases, administering antibiotics under the guidance of a veterinarian.

2. Shell Rot: This condition can result from injuries or bacterial or fungal infections, leading to soft spots or discolored areas on the shell. Treatment includes keeping the shell clean and dry, applying topical treatments, and addressing any underlying infections.

3. Metabolic Bone Disease (MBD): MBD can occur due to a lack of proper UVB lighting, calcium, or vitamin D3, leading to softening of the bones. Treatment involves adjusting the turtle's diet and lighting, providing calcium and vitamin supplements, and consulting a veterinarian for additional care.

4. Parasites: Internal parasites, such as worms and protozoa, can affect a turtle's health, leading to weight loss and diarrhea. Treatment includes deworming medications and maintaining a clean environment to prevent re-infestation.

5. Shell Trauma: Injuries to the shell, such as cracks or breaks, can occur from falls or other traumatic events, and may require cleaning, closure of the wound, and potential supportive care to aid healing.

6. Eye Infections: Symptoms may include swelling, discharge, or difficulty opening the eyes. Treatment involves keeping the eyes clean, using saline solutions to flush the eyes, and consulting a veterinarian if the infection does not improve.

7. Vitamin Deficiencies: Turtles may develop health issues due to a lack of essential vitamins like A, B, or D. Treatment involves adjusting the turtle's diet, using vitamin supplements if necessary, and ensuring proper exposure to UVB light for vitamin D synthesis.

8. Egg Binding: Female turtles may experience difficulty laying eggs, which requires prompt veterinary attention and potential assistance in egg removal if necessary.

9. Intestinal Blockages: Ingestion of foreign objects, such as gravel or plastic, can lead to intestinal blockages. Treatment may involve supportive care, potential surgical intervention, and preventive measures to minimize access to hazardous objects.

10. Mouth rot: Infections or injuries to the mouth can result in inflammation and difficulty eating. Treatment includes oral hygiene, antibiotics, and addressing any underlying causes, such as poor husbandry conditions.

11. Anorexia: Loss of appetite can be a sign of various underlying health issues. Treatment involves identifying and addressing the root cause, providing optimal environmental conditions, and potentially offering enticing food options to encourage feeding.

12. Fungal Infections: Turtles can develop fungal growth on their skin, shell, or in the respiratory tract. Treatment includes antifungal medications, maintaining optimal humidity levels, and ensuring proper hygiene.

13. Salmonella Infections: Turtles are known carriers of Salmonella bacteria, which can pose a risk to human health. Treatment involves strict hygiene practices, regular veterinary check-ups, and minimizing exposure to high-risk individuals, such as young children or individuals with compromised immune systems.

14. Overgrown Beak or Claws: Improper wear of the beak or claws can lead to difficulty eating or moving. Treatment involves regular trimming by a veterinarian familiar with reptiles and providing appropriate substrates for natural wear.

15. Pneumonia: Turtles can develop respiratory infections that affect the lungs and airways. Treatment includes addressing the underlying cause, such as poor environmental conditions or immune system weakness, and incorporating appropriate antibiotics or supportive care to aid recovery.

Pigs

1. Swine Influenza: Symptoms include fever, coughing, nasal discharge, and lethargy. Treatment involves supportive care, rest, and in some cases, antiviral medications prescribed by a veterinarian.

2. Porcine Reproductive and Respiratory Syndrome (PRRS): This viral infection can cause reproductive issues and respiratory problems in pigs. Treatment focuses on supportive care, vaccination, and biosecurity measures to prevent spread.

3. Swine Dysentery: Characterized by bloody diarrhea and weight loss, swine dysentery is treated with antibiotics under the guidance of a veterinarian and strict biosecurity protocols.

4. Foot and Mouth Disease: This highly contagious viral illness requires strict quarantine measures and supportive care, as there is no specific treatment. Prevention through vaccination and biosecurity is essential.

5. Sarcoptic Mange: Caused by mites, sarcoptic mange leads to intense itching and skin lesions. Treatment involves antiparasitic medication, isolating affected animals, and environmental disinfection.

6. Gastric Ulcers: Pigs can develop gastric ulcers from stress, poor diet, or bacterial infection. Treatment includes dietary adjustments, acid-reducing medications, and supportive care.

7. Pneumonia: Respiratory infections in pigs can lead to pneumonia. Treatment involves antibiotics, proper ventilation, and maintaining optimal environmental conditions.

8. Erysipelas: This bacterial infection can cause fever, skin lesions, and arthritis in pigs. Treatment includes antibiotics, vaccination, and isolation of affected animals.

9. Ileitis (Proliferative Enteropathy): A bacterial infection affecting the intestines, ileitis requires antibiotic treatment, dietary management, and stress reduction.

10. Colibacillosis: Escherichia coli infections in pigs can result in diarrhea and systemic illness. Treatment involves antibiotics, supportive care, and focus on hygiene and sanitation.

11. PRRS (Porcine Reproductive and Respiratory Syndrome): This viral respiratory and reproductive disease requires supportive care, vaccination, and biosecurity measures to control spread.

12. Atrophic Rhinitis: This condition can lead to deformities of the pig's snout. Treatment involves vaccination, antibiotic therapy, and, in severe cases, surgical interventions.

13. Prolapse: Reproductive or rectal prolapses require immediate veterinary attention and may require surgical correction or supportive measures such as a pessary to help the affected pig.

14. Mastitis: Inflammation of the udder in lactating sows can lead to mastitis. Treatment includes antibiotic therapy, milking management, and supportive care.

15. Obesity: Overweight pigs can develop various health issues. Treatment involves dietary adjustments, increased physical activity, and monitoring to achieve weight loss.

Monkey

1. Respiratory Infections: Treatment may include antibiotics and supportive care to manage symptoms.

2. Gastrointestinal Disorders: Treatment may involve dietary adjustments, medication to control symptoms, and hydration therapy.

3. Parasitic Infections: Specific antiparasitic medications may be prescribed to treat infestations.

4. Skin Conditions: Treatment may involve topical ointments, medicated baths, or oral medications to manage skin issues.

5. Tuberculosis: This may require a complex treatment plan involving antibiotics and long-term management.

6. Malaria: Antimalarial medications may be considered under the guidance of a veterinarian.

7. Measles: Supportive care, rest, and isolation may be necessary.

8. Hepatitis A: Treatment may focus on supportive therapy and managing symptoms.

9. Simian Immunodeficiency Virus (SIV): There may be ongoing management and supportive care needed for affected monkeys.

10. Ebola: This is a severe and complex illness requiring specialized care and potential quarantine measures.

11. Monkeypox: Treatment may include supportive care, antiviral medications, and isolation.

12. Yellow Fever: Prevention is key, and vaccination may be recommended in affected areas.

13. Salmonellosis: Supportive care, fluid therapy, and antibiotics may be administered.

14. Encephalitis: Treatment may focus on managing symptoms and providing supportive care.

15. Broken Bones or Injuries: Splinting, immobilization, and pain management may be necessary.

Mice

1. Respiratory Infections: Antibiotics and supportive care to manage symptoms such as labored breathing and nasal discharge.

2. Tyzzer's Disease: Treatment may involve antibiotics, supportive care, and hygiene measures to prevent the spread of the disease.

3. Tumors: Surgical removal or palliative care for non-operable cases under the guidance of a veterinarian.

4. Parasitic Infections: Specific antiparasitic medications and environmental sanitation to manage infestations.

5. Overgrown Teeth: Dental care and potential tooth trimming to address malocclusion.

6. Diarrhea and Gastrointestinal Disorders: Dietary adjustments, probiotics, and supportive care to manage digestive issues.

7. Skin Conditions: Treatment may involve topical ointments, medicated baths, or oral medications to manage skin problems.

8. Dehydration: Rehydration therapy and supportive care to address fluid imbalances.

9. Prolapsed Rectum: Manual repositioning and potential surgical intervention if severe.

10. External Injuries: Wound cleaning, pain management, and monitoring for signs of infection.

11. Mites and Lice Infestations: Medications for killing parasites and thorough cleaning of the living environment.

12. Seizures: Identifying underlying causes and potential treatment with medications to control seizures.

13. Neurological Disorders: Treatment may involve diagnostic testing and appropriate medical interventions to manage symptoms.

14. Nutritional Deficiencies: Dietary adjustments and potential supplementation based on identified deficiencies.

Chinchillas

1. Dental Problems: Treatment may involve dental trimming, pain management, and dietary modifications to address overgrowth and malocclusion.

2. Gastrointestinal Stasis: Supportive care, fluid therapy, pain management, and dietary adjustments to manage gut motility issues.

3. Heat Stroke: Immediate cooling measures and supportive care to manage and prevent heat-related illness.

4. Respiratory Infections: Antibiotics, supportive care, and environmental adjustments to manage symptoms like sneezing and labored breathing.

5. Fur Chewing: Identification of underlying causes, environmental enrichment, and potential behavioral interventions under the guidance of a veterinarian.

6. Ear Infections: Antimicrobial medications and ear cleaning to address bacterial or fungal ear infections.

7. Diarrhea and Gastrointestinal Disorders: Dietary adjustments, probiotics, and supportive care to manage digestive issues.

8. Seizures: Identifying underlying causes and potential treatment with medications to control seizures.

9. Skin Conditions: Treatment may involve topical ointments, medicated baths, or oral medications to manage skin issues.

10. Parasitic Infections: Specific antiparasitic medications and environmental disinfection to manage infestations.

11. Obesity: Dietary adjustments, exercise encouragement, and potential weight management strategies.

12. Eye Problems: Ophthalmic medications, eye cleaning, and potential surgical intervention under the guidance of a veterinarian.

13. Urinary Tract Disorders: Antibiotics, dietary adjustments, and supportive care to manage urinary issues.

Gerbils

1. Respiratory Infections: Antibiotics and supportive care to manage symptoms such as sneezing and labored breathing.

2. Diarrhea and Gastrointestinal Disorders: Dietary adjustments, probiotics, and supportive care to manage digestive issues.

3. Dental Problems: Treatment may involve dental trimming, pain management, and dietary modifications.

4. Seizures: Identification of underlying causes and potential treatment with medications to control seizures.

5. Skin Conditions: Treatment may involve topical ointments, medicated baths, or oral medications to manage skin issues.

6. Parasitic Infections: Specific antiparasitic medications may be prescribed to treat infestations.

7. Tumors or Growths: Surgical removal or other appropriate medical interventions under the guidance of a veterinarian.

8. Diabetes: Management may include dietary changes, insulin therapy, and regular monitoring of blood sugar levels.

9. Heatstroke: Immediate cooling measures and supportive care may be needed.

10. Tail Sloughing or Tail Necrosis: Treatment may involve cleaning the affected area, pain management, and possible amputation of the affected part of the tail.

11. Malocclusion (Misalignment of Teeth): Dental care, dietary adjustments, and potential tooth trimming.

12. External Injuries: Treatment may involve wound cleaning, pain management, and monitoring for signs of infection.

13. Nutritional Deficiencies: Dietary adjustments and potential supplementation based on identified deficiencies.

14. Sudden Weight Loss: Identifying underlying causes and addressing any health issues contributing to weight loss.

Rats

1. Respiratory Infections: Antibiotics, supportive care, and environmental adjustments to manage symptoms such as sneezing and labored breathing.

2. Abscesses: Surgical drainage and antibiotic therapy to address localized infections.

3. Tumors: Surgical removal or palliative care for inoperable cases under the guidance of a veterinarian.

4. Parasitic Infections: Specific antiparasitic medications and environmental sanitation to manage infestations such as mites or lice.

5. Diarrhea and Gastrointestinal Disorders: Dietary adjustments, probiotics, and supportive care to manage digestive issues.

6. Malocclusion (Misaligned Teeth): Dental care and potential tooth trimming to address overgrowth and dental problems.

7. Skin Conditions: Treatment may involve topical ointments, medicated baths, or oral medications to manage skin issues.

8. Neurological Disorders: Treatment may involve diagnostic testing and appropriate medical interventions to manage symptoms such as seizures.

9. Dehydration: Rehydration therapy and supportive care to address fluid imbalances.

10. Prolapsed Rectum: Manual repositioning and potential surgical intervention if severe.

11. External Injuries: Wound cleaning, pain management, and monitoring for signs of infection.

12. Ticks and Fleas: Use of appropriate parasiticides and thorough cleaning of the rat's living environment to manage infestations.

13. Endoparasites: Use of anthelmintic medications to treat internal parasites, such as roundworms or hookworms.

14. Reproductive Disorders: Medical or surgical interventions for conditions like uterine tumors or reproductive tract infections.

15. Diet-Related Health Issues: Nutritional adjustments and potential supplementation to manage deficiencies or imbalances.

APPRECIATION

Dear readers,

I want to take a moment to express my heartfelt appreciation for each and every one of you who embarked on the journey through the pages of "Life of a Veterinarian." Your dedication to exploring the world within this novel and your willingness to accompany me on this heartfelt story means more to me than words can express.

When I first set out to write "Life of a Veterinarian," my aim was to shed light on the extraordinary and often overlooked world of veterinary medicine. It was my hope to give readers a glimpse into the joys, challenges, and triumphs that this noble profession entails. Little did I know that the resulting connection and support from all of you would be beyond anything I could have imagined.

To all the aspiring veterinarians who have found solace and reassurance within the pages of this novel, I want to commend you for your tremendous dedication to animal welfare. Your passion for making a difference in the lives of our furry friends is truly inspiring, and I am honored to be a part of your journey.

Lastly, I would like to extend my deepest appreciation to those readers who may not have a direct connection to the field of veterinary medicine, yet embraced this story with open hearts. Your willingness to explore new worlds and gain insight into the experiences of others is a testament to your empathy and open-mindedness. Thank you for allowing me to take you on this unforgettable adventure.

It is with immense gratitude that I sign off, knowing that "Life of a Veterinarian" has found a place in your hearts. Your support has been a constant reminder that stories have the power to transport us, to teach us, and to unite us in ways that we may never fully comprehend. It is the readers like you who reinforce my belief in the transformative power of literature and reaffirm my dedication to sharing stories that inspire, uplift, and educate.

As I reflect on this incredible journey, I am reminded of the saying, "A book is only as good as its readers." And in the case of "Life of a Veterinarian," I am beyond grateful for the extraordinary readership that has embraced this book with open arms and open minds. Your continued support, word-of-mouth recommendations, and heartfelt discussions have made this novel more than just a collection of words on paper – it has become a shared experience, a community of individuals bound together by a love for storytelling.

To express my gratitude, I am committed to continuing my work as an author, striving to bring you more stories that capture your hearts, challenge your perspectives, and uplift your spirits.

Your dedication as readers inspires me to delve deeper, to research more extensively, and to write with greater empathy. It is my hope that through all my future works, I can continue to touch your lives in meaningful ways.

Whether you laughed, cried, or pondered the deeper themes within "Life of a Veterinarian," please know that your presence has made a lasting impact on me as an author. I genuinely appreciate the time and energy you have invested in reading this novel and immersing yourself in its narrative. Your commitment to literature and your engagement with this story validate the countless hours poured into its creation.

Once again, I extend my heartfelt appreciation to all of you, dear readers, for your unwavering support, kindness, and understanding. Thank you for playing such an essential role in bringing "Life of a Veterinarian" to life, and for being a part of this incredible literary journey. It is a privilege to have you by my side as we venture into the vast world of storytelling together.

As you have the intrest of your animals in heat make sure you make them feel loved and take proper care of them. Do not neglect any signs you notice in your animals.

With sincere gratitude,

Merit Nicholas (Author of "Life of a Veterinarian")

www.ingramcontent.com/pod-product-compliance
Lightning Source LLC
Chambersburg PA
CBHW040319220526
45473CB00009B/2498